Adolescent Public Mental Health

Patricia Gail Bray • Arthur Maerlender
Editors

Adolescent Public Mental Health

Why Systems Need Changing and How a Public Mental Health Approach Can Work

Springer

Editors
Patricia Gail Bray
Department of Management, Policy and Community Health, UTHealth Houston School of Public Health
The University of Texas Health Science Center (UTHealth) at Houston
Houston, TX, USA

Arthur Maerlender
Department of Psychology
Saint Anselm College
Manchester, NH, USA

Center for Brain, Biology and Behavior
University of Nebraska
Lincoln, NE, USA

ISBN 978-3-031-68293-3 ISBN 978-3-031-68294-0 (eBook)
https://doi.org/10.1007/978-3-031-68294-0

This Springer imprint is published by the registered company Springer Nature Switzerland AG
The registered company address is: Gewerbestrasse 11, 6330 Cham, Switzerland

For Stephen.
Patricia Gail Bray

For global youth: do better than we did.
Arthur Maerlender

Foreword

Mental health has been the focus of The Menninger Clinic's mission since 1925. From almost the beginning, our organization has been tending to the mental wellness of children and adolescents, including research and treatment beginning with operation in Topeka, Kansas, continuing with our move to Houston, Texas, in 2003.

Menninger's focus on adolescent mental health received a momentous boost with the generous $7.5 million in support from the David and Helen Gurley Brown Trust, now the Helen Gurley Brown Foundation, in 2015. Under the direction of this book's co-editor, Patricia Gail Bray, Menninger launched an adolescent mental health initiative to address the emerging adolescent mental health crisis. Our public educators, as well as the nonprofits providing support, revealed there was a desperate need for a social and emotional learning (SEL) approach, especially in underserved and culturally diverse populations of Greater Houston, Texas. Dr. Bray worked with the Foundation to initiate and oversee the formulation of the BridgeUp Model to support schoolwide SEL programs, behavioral health supports, and collaboration. The overall purpose was for schools, the community, and families to nurture the whole child to increase the likelihood of remaining in school and graduating while utilizing the SEL tools that buoyed their well-being.

Dr. Bray and her editorial colleague, Dr. Arthur Maerlender, made certain to track the progress of the 63,325 Greater Houston students who participated in BridgeUp programming. Once I joined The Menninger Clinic as President and CEO in 2019, the students who showed signs of stress-related difficulties with attendance, scholastic work, or behavioral issues were already being identified early through the participants' multi-tiered system of support. Menninger and other mental health treatment providers ensured that the students who needed mental health treatment received the necessary treatment services.

As you will see spotlighted in this book, one of the BridgeUp students who came to The Menninger Clinic for treatment was JoJo. She illustrates why this model is needed and how this model works when it's implemented. JoJo's situation also is an example of the value of applying this adolescent public health initiative nationwide.

As the U.S. Surgeon General Dr. Vivek H. Murthy has pointed out, America is overdue for integrating mental health into the public health sphere. I wholeheartedly agree with the co-editors that collaboration holds the key for solving the multifaceted issues facing today's adolescents. Their Adolescent Public Mental Health (APMH) model outlined was born out of the BridgeUp experience in Houston, the nation's fourth most populous metropolitan area. Regardless of the size of public-school districts, and also private schools, collaboration is an essential element in achieving success with a critical public health initiative.

Mentally healthy adolescents will equate to healthier families and flourishing communities.

It has been my pleasure as a colleague of Dr. Bray to be a witness to the transformation in our communities, including:

- More adolescents believing someone at school cares about them
- Academic scores improving
- Disciplinary referrals declining
- Student suicides decreasing
- Families learning to support their students

Here at The Menninger Clinic, we are acutely aware that many parents and decision makers may not recognize that half of mental health challenges emerge by the age of 14 years. We are working to reduce the stigma surrounding mental health issues, which, ironically, many adolescents and young people found it essential to express during the pandemic. Residual isolation and missed adolescent rites of passage continue to exacerbate the mental health in the adolescent population today, which is why this book is so timely.

Utilizing our family, academic, and community systems is as essential to realizing the editors' vision to turn around the declining adolescent mental health crisis. Only if we start with a proven solution will America make a positive difference in overall health and mental health for generations.

President and CEO, The Menninger Clinic Armando E. Colombo
Houston, TX, USA

Preface

During the 1990s, Dr. M. David Low was the President of The University of Texas Health Science Center (UTHealth Houston). Born in Alberta, Canada, he received his MD from Queens College in Canada and a PhD from Baylor College of Medicine in Houston, Texas. His expertise and experience bridged medicine and public health. He brought this unique perspective to his service as a founding board member of a new philanthropic arm of the St. Luke's Episcopal Health System. The St. Luke's Episcopal Health Charities (Charities) was located in the Texas Medical Center, home to 49 nonprofit health organizations, including UTHealth Houston and Baylor College of Medicine.

The principal editor of this book had the fortunate experience to work closely with Dr. Low during that time. What he brought to the table changed the face of public health and philanthropy in southeast Texas. Dr. Low, always a teacher, freely shared the knowledge gleaned from his vast experience, including his many years of collaborative partnerships with the Canadian Institute for Advanced Research (CIFAR) and University College London (UCL).

Many of his CIFAR and UCL colleagues represented some of the best minds in the emerging Social Determinants of Health (SDOH) research and its application specifically to addressing health inequities. The timing could not have been better for our charitable organization. Dr. Low introduced the Charities' team to many of these researchers. The result was cutting-edge research and approaches that helped to guide the funding of almost $100 million in community-based interventions in 57 southeastern Texas counties, covering 40% of the state's population.

This current volume would not be possible without Dr. Low's early guidance and that of the CIFAR and UCL researchers leading social determinants of health research. These scholars gave generously of their time and knowledge to our Charities' team, and indirectly to BridgeUp at Menninger, the focus of this book, which helped to transform the lives of 63,325 underserved adolescents in the Houston metropolitan area during 2015–2022. The roots of BridgeUp are found in his willingness to serve on a new philanthropic community board and to share his experience.

To our knowledge, during this time, there were few US organizations implementing an SDOH approach in public health or mental health research or practice. After the U.S. Surgeon General declared a youth mental health crisis in 2021, the American Psychiatric Association formally approved legislation and policies in March 2022 to recognize the relationship of SDOH with mental health, well-being, and equity.[1] The adoption of SDOH, together with prevention, results in a public health approach and is one of the defining features of an innovative Adolescent Public Mental Health (APMH) model, proposed in this volume. The BridgeUp Case Study serves as the basis for the development of the APMH model.

The purpose of the BridgeUp Model was to improve adolescent mental health in some of the most underserved areas of Houston. Most of the 46 BridgeUp interventions were implemented in secondary schools. Two years after the project ended, three independent school districts have sustained the model beyond the duration of the BridgeUp project, reaching approximately 72,105 students, surpassing the number reached during the project. The potential reach and sustainability of the demonstration project is the motivation for this volume, including the science behind its success and a brief review of similar initiatives taking place in other countries around the world.

Houston, TX, USA — Patricia Gail Bray
Manchester, NH, USA — Arthur Maerlender

[1] The American Psychiatric Association. (2022, March). Report of the Presidential Task Force on Social Determinants of Mental Health. Retrieved April 10, 2024, from https://www.psychiatry.org/getmedia/3f7df9f3-2c59-4b12-b551-a776cce09ddb/2022-APA-TFSDMH-Board-of-Trustees-March-Report.pdf

About Adolescent Public Mental Health

This book advocates for an innovative public mental health model designed to address a pressing issue—the declining mental health of adolescents globally and in the United States. Public mental health is an emerging field that involves a population approach to mental health, and includes prevention and treatment of mental disorders, prevention of associated impacts, and promotion of mental well-being in school settings, including for those recovering from mental disorders.[1] Essentially, a public health approach is adopted to enhance adolescent mental health, drawing on concepts from three core systems: public health, mental health, and school mental health. The inspiration for this book arose from the impactful experiences in creating and managing such a program.

Over a seven-year period, a novel public mental health model was developed and implemented at the David and Helen Gurley Brown BridgeUp: Mental Health Center (BridgeUp) at The Menninger Clinic in Houston, Texas—a leading mental health system in the United States. This initiative serves as the case study for the book. The multisector approach employed was anchored in systems change, public health research and practice, and with the specific aim to improve adolescent mental health.

Despite scholarly and public media attention to post-pandemic declines in adolescent mental health, few published sources present a sustainable, scalable, and collaborative solution that integrates attention to the social determinants of health, equity, and prevention with mental health literacy education, early intervention, and collective impact. To our knowledge, there hasn't been a replicable model implemented on the same scale as BridgeUp. Globally, however, there are many promising, systems-level exemplars emerging. A sampling is included in this volume.

While it is known that prevention, combined with diagnosis and treatment, is the most effective way to address disease, mental health promotion and mental illness prevention have been slower to gain traction, when compared to cardiovascular

[1] Campion, J. (2018). Public mental health: Key challenges and opportunities. *BJPsych International. 3*, 51–54.

disease and cancer. This is changing with increased intersections among the core systems of adolescent mental health, public health, and school health. The integrative approach has only recently emerged in the applied scientific literature. Vice Admiral, Vivek H. Murthy, U.S. Surgeon General, is altering the dialogue, opening up more channels of communication to address the adolescent mental health crisis in relation to population health. The "calls to action" included in this book consist of 24 recommendations relevant for leaders in public health, mental health, and education, aligning with this changing national and global conversation.

Acknowledgments

We would like to thank the thousands of adolescents, teachers, administrators, schools, nonprofit leaders, mental health providers, BridgeUp program directors, and advisory committee volunteers who helped to ensure that the BridgeUp at Menninger project was a success. This project and book would not be possible without their extraordinary efforts.

We are indebted to the Helen Gurley Brown Foundation's Eve Burton, Kim St. Clair-Boden, and Roger Paschke and their generous funding to The Menninger Clinic. The funding provided the means to create the David and Helen Gurley Brown BridgeUp: Mental Health Center (BridgeUp). At this center, an innovative adolescent public mental health model was created and implemented throughout the Houston metropolitan area for 7 years. The inspiration and motivation for this volume came from that work. Many extraordinary individuals from Menninger played significant roles, and for their commitment and dedication to BridgeUp, we thank them. Special thanks to Armando Colombo, Stephanie Cunningham, Tony Gaglio, Jon Stevens, Megan Kale, Linda Jones, Nancy Corbet, Nancy Trowbridge, Ed Coffey, Jennifer O'Bryant, Summer Bartlett-Moore, Anissa Orr, Jewel Stevens, Kevin Harwerth, Martin Acuna, Cherri Carbonara, and Kristin Taylor Strauder.

The BridgeUp leadership team made substantive contributions to the design, development, implementation, and evaluation. We are grateful for the leadership of Linda Civallero, Robert Wimpelberg, Oana Pop, Isabella Acuna, and the other Brown Fellows. Additionally, the success of the project was possible because of in-kind support from the Menninger Board, the Foundation Board, and the Menninger philanthropy, marketing, finance, security, IT, and food services departments. We also thank the generous support from our donors, especially from Flo McGee with the McGee Family Foundation.

We thank Robert K. Wimpelberg, Donna Lord Black, and Oana Smaranda Pop for their scholarly contributions to this volume.

Many other friends and colleagues have contributed in countless ways, including Danna Kurtin, Susan Fordice, Tim Garson, Jean Raphael, Wendy Ward, Christine Adams, Jackie Flores, Janet Pozmantier, Jane Mahoney, Kay York, Teresa Southwell, Mukund Nair, Elizabeth Holbrook, Carla Cooper, and M. David Low.

The Springer staff has provided invaluable support, and we would like to give special thanks to Janet Kim, Kausalya Boobalan, and Richard Lansing.

Heartfelt thanks to our families who have given much to help this project come to fruition. With their support, we hope to continue impacting the lives of the many adolescents we have worked with, and for those who follow.

Contents

About the Contributors

Donna Lord Black, MA is a distinguished published author, school practitioner, policy leader, and an education advocate. She has 30 years of career and professional growth and experience. As a dually licensed professional, she holds expertise in both school and clinical psychology. Through an extensive network of professional connections, she has earned commendable recognition for her unwavering moral and ethical character. Her contributions and service to the profession have been recognized at the state and national levels and she is both honored and privileged to serve as a catalyst for positive change in the profession. She received her Master of Arts in Clinical Psychology from the University of Houston-Clear Lake in Texas.

Oana Smaranda Pop, MPH was a Brown Fellow with the BridgeUp Center at The Menninger Clinic between 2018 and 2020. She conducted research on barriers, evaluation, and stakeholder engagement for the program, and provided administrative support. She has a Bachelor of Arts in Integrative Biology from the University of California, Berkeley, a Master of Public Health in Community Health Practice, and a Certificate in Health Disparities from the University of Texas Health Science Center at Houston, School of Public Health. She now works as a health informatics specialist.

Robert K. Wimpelberg, PhD is the Founder and Executive Director of All Kids Alliance at the University of Houston, Texas, where he is Professor Emeritus and former Dean of the College of Education. After 20 years in university administration and more than 50 years in education, he dedicates his encore career to working with organizations interested in collective impact, collaborative action, and continuous quality improvement. He graduated from Yale University, and following doctoral work at the University of Chicago, he joined the faculty at Tulane University and later moved to the University of New Orleans in Louisiana.

Contributors

Patricia Gail Bray Department of Management, Policy and Community Health, UTHealth Houston School of Public Health, The University of Texas Health Science Center (UTHealth) at Houston, Houston, TX, USA

Arthur Maerlender Department of Psychology, Saint Anselm College, Manchester, NH, USA

Center for Brain, Biology and Behavior, University of Nebraska—Lincoln, Lincoln, NE, USA

Donna Lord Black Independent Educational Consultant, Frisco, TX, USA

Social-Emotional Learning Alliance for Texas (SEL4TX.org), Frisco, TX, USA

Academy for Social-Emotional Learning in Schools, Rutgers University, New Brunswick, NJ, USA

Oana Smaranda Pop Independent Researcher, Houston, TX, USA

Robert K. Wimpelberg All Kids Alliance, College of Education, University of Houston, Houston, TX, USA

About the Editors

Patricia Gail Bray, PhD is a dedicated public health and nonprofit executive deeply committed to fostering systems and social change, equity, and research-informed multidisciplinary initiatives, specifically with marginalized populations. She holds an adjunct appointment at UTHealth Houston's School of Public Health in Texas and is president of Westlake Health Consulting, LLC. Her extensive expertise includes applying scientific methodologies to co-developing and scaling complex collaborative programs and models at the intersection of medicine and public health. She has 30 years of experience working with the Texas Medical Center healthcare systems, including 7 years at The Menninger Clinic. She received her Public Health doctoral degree from UTHealth Houston's School of Public Health.

Arthur Maerlender, PhD, ABPP-CN is Board Certified in Clinical Neuropsychology, a Research Associate Professor at the Center for Brain, Biology and Behavior at the University of Nebraska and Adjunct Professor at the University of Nebraska Medical Center in the Department of Neurological Sciences. Additionally, he is an Associate Professor and Senior Research Fellow in the Department of Psychology at Saint Anselm College in New Hampshire. He has worked with Dr. Bray for the past 8 years, advising and mentoring her work at Menninger. Currently, he is an integral voice for the important intersection between mental health, education, and public health. He received his doctoral degree from the University of Notre Dame in Counseling Psychology.

Abbreviations

AACAP	American Academy of Child and Adolescent Psychiatry
AAP	American Academy of Pediatrics
ABC	American Broadcasting System
AC	Advisory Committee for BridgeUp
ACA	Affordable Care Act
ACE	Adverse Childhood Experiences
AHRQ	Agency for Healthcare Research and Quality
AIR	American Institutes for Research
AMA	American Medical Association
AMH	Adolescent Mental Health
APHA	American Public Health Association
APMH	Adolescent Public Mental Health
ASCD	Association for Supervision and Curriculum Development
AWARE	Advancing Wellness and Resilience in Education
CAHPS	Consumer Assessment of Healthcare Providers and Systems
CASEL	Collaborative for Academic, Social and, Emotional Learning
CCSSO	Council of Chief State School Officers
CDC	Centers for Disease Control and Prevention
CEO	Chief Executive Officer
CHA	Children's Hospital Association
CHIP	Children's Health Insurance Program
CI	Collective Impact
CIFAR	The Canadian Institute for Advanced Research
CMD	Common Mental Disorders
CNS	Central Nervous System
COVID-19	Coronavirus Disease 2019
CP	Critical Periods
DALY	Disability-Adjusted Life Years
DDDM	Data-Driven Decision-Making
DSM	Diagnostic and Statistical Manual of Mental Disorders
EAHCA or EHA	Education for All Handicapped Children Act

EDs	Editors
EGM	Evidence and Gap Map
ELS	Early Life Stressors
ESEA	Elementary and Secondary Education Act
ESSA	Every Student Succeeds Act
ESSER	Elementary and Secondary School Emergency Relief
FAPE	Free and Appropriate Public Education
GHQ	General Health Questionnaire
HGB	Helen Gurley Brown Foundation
HHS	Health and Human Services
HPSA	Health Professional Shortage Area
IDEA	Individuals with Disabilities Education Act
IDEIA	Individuals with Disabilities Educational Improvement Act
IOM	Institute of Medicine (Changed names in 2015 to The National Academy of Medicine)
ISD	Independent School District
KPI	Key Performance Indicators
LEA	Local Education Agency
LM	Logic Models
MDD	Major Depressive Disorder
MDE	Major Depressive Episode
MHPSS	Mental Health and Psychosocial Support
MHQ	Mental Health Quotient
MOU	Memoranda of Understanding
MRI	Magnetic Resonance Imaging
MTSS	Multi-Tiered System of Supports
NAM	The National Academy of Medicine
NAS	The National Academies of Sciences, Engineering, and Medicine
NASP	National Association of School Psychologists
NCLB	The No Child Left Behind Act of 2001
NCSMH	National Center for School Mental Health
NIH	National Institutes of Health
NIMH	National Institutes of Mental Health
NPP	Negative Predictive Power
OECD	Organisation for Economic Co-operation and Development
PBIS	Positive Behavioral Interventions and Support
PFC	Prefrontal Cortical Circuits
PHQ-9	Patient Health Questionnaire-9
PHS	Public Health Services
PPV	Positive Predictive Power
PSC	Pediatric System Checklist
PTSD	Post-Traumatic Stress Disorder
PV	Parvalbumin-Positive
RCI	Rapid Cycle Improvement

RCT	Randomized Clinical Trial
RFP	Request for Proposal
RTI	Response to Intervention
SAMHSA	Substance Abuse Mental Health Services Administration
SDOH	Social Determinants of Health
SDOMH	Social Determinants of Mental Health
SE	Social-Ecological
SEA	State Education Agency
SEL	Social, Emotional Learning
SLD	Specific Learning Disabilities
SMART	Specific, Measurable, Achievable, Relevant, and Time-Bound Goals
SUD	Substance Use Disorders
SWPBIS	Schoolwide Positive Behavioral Interventions and Supports
TANF	Temporary Assistance for Needy Families
TMC	The Texas Medical Center
ToC	Theory of Change
U.K.	United Kingdom
U.S.	The United States
UCL	University College London
UCLA	University of California, Los Angeles
UNESCO	United Nations Educational, Scientific and Cultural Organization
UNICEF	United Nations Children's Fund
WHO	World Health Organization
WM	Working Memory
WSCC	Whole School, Whole Community, Whole Child
YRBSS	Youth Risk Behavior Surveillance Survey

List of Figures

List of Tables

Chapter 1
Introduction to Adolescent Public Mental Health

Patricia Gail Bray and Arthur Maerlender

1.1 Introduction

The premise of this volume is that healthy adolescent development is critical for the near-term future of the population. As such, like other important periods of development (i.e., infants 0–3 years old), adolescence deserves focused attention and nurturance that does not currently exist at a system level. Thus, in support of the science of human development, a new focus, a systems change is called for to provide improved pathways for fostering the recognition and support of adolescent mental health (AMH) (WHO, 2002). As part of the systems change, a new model called *adolescent public mental health* is proposed and is based on a compelling 7-year demonstration project in Houston, Texas. Adding urgency to this call is the fact of an ongoing, global crisis in AMH. This crisis has been acknowledged and declared by several USA government and professional organizations (AAP, 2021).

Although the pandemic may be the proximal event that has cast a spotlight on the AMH problem, the reality of declining adolescent mental health was being reported long before COVID-19. Prevalence rates of adolescents with depression, anxiety, self-harm, and suicide all increased before, during, and after the pandemic (Agency for Healthcare Research and Quality (US), 2022).

P. G. Bray (✉)
Department of Management, Policy and Community Health, UTHealth Houston School of Public Health, The University of Texas Health Science Center (UTHealth) at Houston, Houston, TX, USA
e-mail: Patricia.G.Bray@uth.tmc.edu

A. Maerlender
Department of Psychology, Saint Anselm College, Manchester, NH, USA

Center for Brain, Biology and Behavior, University of Nebraska—Lincoln, Lincoln, NE, USA
e-mail: amaerlender@anselm.edu

P. G. Bray, A. Maerlender (eds.), *Adolescent Public Mental Health*,
https://doi.org/10.1007/978-3-031-68294-0_1

On a positive note, since the pandemic, there has been more research focused on adolescent mental health and the implementation of innovative programs. This has resulted in an increase in the range of solutions, both in the USA and globally. Yet the seemingly intractable AMH crisis continues to elude scalable and sustainable corrections. Based on the complex, multifactorial reasons that can cause significant increased adverse impacts on adolescents and potentially cause fewer protective effects, the solutions put forward to address the AMH crisis should also be multifactorial, addressing the required complexity.

This volume argues for a systems change approach that seeks to address multiple layers that separately and collectively end up supporting the current unsatisfactory status quo. By invoking multiple interpersonal and societal elements and implementing evidence-based programs, the goal is to instantiate a systems approach to improving adolescent outcomes by implementing an *adolescent public mental health* (APMH) model.

However, creating new and innovative systems necessarily addresses influential contextual factors such as culture, existing institutions, schools and organizations, and political and social factors. Thus, a successful public health approach to adolescent mental health would involve the integration of concepts, organizations, and services at different levels of the social structure. These would include public health promotion, prevention, and monitoring strategies together with the understanding of local social determinants of health. Additional levels include the use of existing mental health services, leveraging the role and resources of the public education system, and respecting the history of successes and failures in the receiving community. Fortunately, implementation science provides guidance for addressing the barriers inherent in the multiple application of evidence-based innovations (Bauer & Kirchner, 2020).

The chapters address the rationale for the systems change needed, strategies and tools for making sustainable change happen, and an example of one evidence-based project that successfully implemented these concepts and approaches. Based on the project, a new APMH model is proposed as a possible roadmap with the purpose of improving adolescent mental health.

1.2 Structure and Contents of the Volume

The volume is organized into two parts. The first part is a justification about *why* an adolescent systems change is needed. Part I "*Why* Adolescent Mental Health Needs a Systems Change" includes Chaps. 2, 3, and 4. The second part is an example about how to implement, scale, and sustain a systems change with a new adolescent public mental health model. Part II is "*How* to Make a Systems Change for Adolescent Mental Health" and includes Chaps. 5, 6, 7, 8, 9, 10, and 11.

1.2.1 Part I: Why *Adolescent Mental Health Needs a Systems Change*

Part I presents a high level overview of the adolescent mental health system, focusing on the state of adolescence in the twenty-first century and the interconnections to school mental health and public health. The complexity of the challenges and the continued intractability to address those challenges is presented. The final chapter in Part I includes a justification and an argument for *why* a systems change is needed in adolescent mental health and introduces a full discussion of the APMH model.

1.2.2 Chapter 2: Adolescent Mental Health in the Twenty-First Century

The state of adolescence is examined through a biopsychosocial-cultural lens. This view marks a shift in the literature of adolescent mental health to become more holistic, equitable, and integrated with the social, family, school, and community influences. Neurobiological underpinnings at the most basic level, and environmental influences, called the *social determinants of health*, at the other end of the human continuum are also acknowledged. This chapter also takes issue with the terminologies of mental health, mental illness, and well-being, arguing that a focus on well-being is the more parsimonious approach to population stability.

1.2.3 Chapter 3: School Mental Health Milestones Since the Late Twentieth Century

Chapter 3 emphasizes the role of public secondary schools responding to the mental health needs of adolescents as a means to support mental wellness. The evolving school mental health system is reviewed and makes the argument that public schools are identified as optimal environments for designing and implementing effective public health interventions for this age group (Black, 2022). The twenty-first century interplay between secondary schools and health within the USA education system is explored, with an emphasis on building developmentally supportive school organizations to cultivate healthy and productive adolescents. School governance, connectedness practices, school health policies, and the professions necessary to enhance adolescent mental health within school settings are also reviewed.

1.2.4 Chapter 4: Systems Change: Constructing an Adolescent Public Mental Health Model

Drawing on research supporting a public health approach to mental health forms the basis for systems change in adolescent mental health. The acknowledgement and interconnectivity of the public health, adolescent mental health, and school health systems helps to support and justify why a systems change is needed at both the individual and population levels of adolescent mental health. The unique interdependency of these systems suggests a new model, APMH, to address adolescent mental health more holistically.

1.3 Part II: *How* to Make a Systems Change for Adolescent Mental Health

Part II presents chapters focused on *how* a systems change approach to an adolescent public mental health model can be implemented to result in optimal adolescent mental health and well-being. The strategies necessary to implement a successful case study are introduced and reviewed. The case study, along with other global models with similar themes, demonstrates that potential solutions to the AMH crisis are possible and are, in part, underway. Building on the research, many elements of a new APMH model already exists. The next three chapters explore in more detail lessons with model implementation in a multisystems environment, the equity challenges regarding mental health access to care, and the importance of adolescent public mental health screening. The book concludes with a summary of necessary next steps for taking action with an APMH model.

1.3.1 Chapter 5: Strategies for Implementing a Public Health Model for Adolescent Mental Health

This chapter explores how the conceptual background theory sets the stage for systems change with the implementation of an adolescent public mental health model. A macro-level effort is needed that integrates mental health, public health, schools, and communities with theory-based governance and management structures. Examples of these structures include implementation science, collective impact and theory of change, among others, providing clarity for mapping a comprehensive implementation plan.

1.3.2 Chapter 6: The BridgeUp Case Study: The BridgeUp Model Implementations

The BridgeUp case study in this chapter reviews the design, development, and implementation for the pilot model used in the demonstration project. The school-based implementation of a public health approach to adolescent mental health is discussed together with strategies for addressing poverty, education, and other social determinants of health (SDOH). A particular focus on equity issues that differentially impact vulnerable adolescents in underserved areas is discussed (Gorski & Landsman, 2014). The case study highlights the value of a *public health approach*, which includes mental health promotion, prevention, and the SDOH. Multisector partnerships are comprised of key stakeholders from multiple school districts and mental health providers located in the Houston, Texas area.

1.3.3 Chapter 7: Global Adolescent Mental Health

Chapter 7 presents a brief overview of global progress regarding the core systems of adolescent mental health. Highlights of other countries reveal advancements to help adapt and adopt a global adolescent public mental health model. Consideration of the differences in resources is reviewed with an informative analysis across lower and higher income countries.

1.3.4 Chapter 8: Lessons Part 1: Lessons, Limitations, and Funding of the BridgeUp Model

The culmination of the challenges, successes, and limitations learned from the BridgeUp demonstration project is presented. These learnings are applicable to the proposed APMH model. Additionally, the challenges and successes about how to plan for model scalability and sustainability are discussed. Steps to guide action are outlined together with strategies, tactics, and leadership for managing programs across multiple sites and partners. Such an effort requires a reconceptualization of the functions and roles of the related systems.

1.3.5 Chapter 9: Lessons Part 2: Barriers to Care

Inequities in mental health is a theme that is addressed and integrated with the APMH model. This chapter features an overview of the nine distinctive barriers to mental healthcare for adolescents. Proposed next steps are discussed with the goal of including approaches to reduce these barriers for adolescent mental health in the future.

1.3.6 Chapter 10: Lessons Part 3: Public Mental Health Screening for Adolescents

This chapter takes a public health approach regarding mental health screening for adolescents. The risks, benefits, and costs of screening are discussed, including psychometric adequacy. Effective screening can enhance the implementation of mental health promotion and prevention strategies, as well as address equity implications, which can provide benefit to adolescents as well as the entire community.

1.3.7 Chapter 11: Taking Action with the Adolescent Public Mental Health Model

The key themes inherent in the adolescent public mental health model are summarized and serve as the basis for how to reframe possible approaches to enhance adolescent mental health. Utilizing the National Center for Safe, Supportive Learning's (n.d.) rubric for school mental health, six recommendations for implementation of the APMH model are outlined. To conclude the volume, 24 recommendations are offered as a roadmap to improve adolescent mental health in the USA and globally.

1.4 Conclusion

Together with system-level procedures such as implementation science, a collective impact framework and a theory of change approach, a sea change in producing more effective and sustainable systems and programs can be established across a wide array of social and mental health-related problems. Leveraging empirical evidence and the firsthand experience of implementing an adolescent public mental health program, this volume provides a rationale for a public health approach with an adolescent public mental health model.

Competing Interests

1. *The BridgeUp at Menninger study was generously funded by the David and Helen Gurley Brown Trust, BridgeUp: Mental Health at The Menninger Clinic.*
2. Patricia Gail Bray *has received consultant fees from* The Menninger Clinic, located in Houston, Texas.

References

Agency for Healthcare Research and Quality (U.S.). (2022). *National healthcare quality and disparities report*. Rockville, MD. Retrieved March 30, 2024, from https://www.ncbi.nlm.nih.gov/books/NBK587174/

American Academy of Pediatrics (AAP). (2021). *Declaration of a national emergency in child and adolescent mental health*. Retrieved January 25, 2023, from https://www.aap.org/en/advocacy/child-and-adolescent-healthy-mental-development/aap-aacap-cha-declaration-of-a-national-emergency-in-child-and-adolescent-mental-health/

Bauer, M. S., & Kirchner, J. (2020). Implementation science: What is it and why should I care? *Psychiatry Research, 283*, 112376. https://doi.org/10.1016/j.psychres.2019.04.025

Black, D. (2022). *Essentials of social emotional learning (SEL): The complete guide for schools and practitioners* (A. Kaufman & N. Kaufman, Eds.). Wiley.

Gorski, P. C., & Landsman, J. (2014). *The poverty and education reader: A call for equity in many voices* (1st ed.). Routledge. https://www.routledge.com/The-Poverty-and-Education-Reader-A-Call-for-Equity-in-Many-Voices/Gorski-Landsman/p/book/9781579228590

National Center for Safe, Supportive Learning Environments (NCSSF) (n.d.). *Implementing school mental health supports: Best practices in action*. Retrieved March 30, 2024, from https://safesupportivelearning.ed.gov/sites/default/files/13-ImpSchMnHlthSprtBtPrt-508_0.pdf

World Health Organization (WHO). (2002). *Adolescent friendly health services: An agenda for change*. Retrieved January 20, 2024, from https://iris.who.int/bitstream/handle/10665/67923/WHO_FCH_CAH_02.14.pdf

Part I
Why Adolescent Mental Health Needs a Systems Change

Chapter 2
Adolescent Mental Health in the Twenty-First Century

Arthur Maerlender and Patricia Gail Bray

2.1 Introduction

Due to the effects of global and local catastrophes including the COVID-19 pandemic, ongoing wars, mass shootings, and climate change, there can be little doubt that worldwide mental health is experiencing a difficult point in time (Protecting Youth Mental Health: The U.S. Surgeon General's Advisory, 2021; Clark et al., 2021). Exposed to cultural change during an important developmental stage of life, adolescents may suffer the most cognitively, socially, and psychologically in times of cultural stress. Further, the negative effect on their development bodes ill for the next generation of parents and leaders. This chapter provides a brief history of adolescent healthcare which includes current demographics and an overview of brain development theories and research. It then examines the scope of the crisis by discussing adolescent suicide, post-traumatic stress disorder, and anxiety. Coping strategies, both healthy and unhealthy, are included in this overview.

The World Health Organization (WHO) defines an adolescent as any person between the ages of 10 and 19. As a transitional phase of growth between childhood and adulthood, it is a critical developmental stage which changes in real

A. Maerlender (✉)
Department of Psychology, Saint Anselm College, Manchester, NH, USA

Center for Brain, Biology and Behavior, University of Nebraska—Lincoln, Lincoln, NE, USA
e-mail: amaerlender@anselm.edu; amaerlender2@unl.edu

P. G. Bray
Department of Management, Policy and Community Health, UTHealth Houston School of Public Health, The University of Texas Health Science Center (UTHealth) at Houston, Houston, TX, USA
e-mail: Patricia.G.Bray@uth.tmc.edu

P. G. Bray, A. Maerlender (eds.), *Adolescent Public Mental Health*,
https://doi.org/10.1007/978-3-031-68294-0_2

time. Further, today's exposures, risks, and pressures are quantitatively different for adolescents from those of their parents and thus create unique challenges, especially considering the adolescent system of care. Adolescents have traditionally obtained clinical services, including those for mental health, through pediatrics or, if older, through adult services. It was not until 1988 that the American Academy of Child Psychiatry added "Adolescent" to its title (American Academy of Child and Adolescent Psychiatry, n.d.). By placing it within child psychiatry, however, they did not provide specialized, differentiated training (Barthel, 2007). And it was not until 2002 that the WHO called for an agenda of change and the subspecialty of adolescent medicine was formally adopted (Lee et al., 2016; WHO, 2002).

2.2 A Brief Timeline of US Adolescent Care

Adolescence has not been a consistently defined or characterized developmental period, and the community perception of adolescence has changed over time. In terms of adolescent health, there have been significant changes and advancements over the course of the nineteenth, twentieth, and twenty-first centuries. Several factors have influenced these changes, including advancements in medical science, improvements in public health infrastructure, changes in social and cultural norms, and the development of healthcare policies and programs.

A brief timeline of these changes reveals increasing importance given to this period of development within the context of significant change over time.

2.2.1 *Nineteenth Century*

- Limited understanding: During the nineteenth century, medical knowledge and understanding of adolescent health were relatively limited. Many diseases and health conditions that affected adolescents were poorly understood, and treatment options were often rudimentary.
- High mortality rates: Infectious diseases, malnutrition, and lack of access to healthcare contributed to high mortality rates among adolescents during this period. The average life expectancy in 1860 was about half of what it is today (O'Neill, n.d.).
- Lack of preventive measures: Preventive measures, such as vaccination and sanitation practices, were not widely available, leading to the spread of communicable diseases.
- Minimal formal education: Education about health and hygiene was limited, and formal schooling for adolescents was not universally accessible.

2.2.2 Twentieth Century

- Advances in medicine: The twentieth century witnessed significant advances in medical science, leading to the discovery of antibiotics and vaccines that greatly reduced the impact of infectious diseases on adolescents.
- Public health interventions: The establishment of public health measures, including immunization campaigns and sanitation improvements, contributed to improved overall health for adolescents.
- Focus on education: The importance of education for adolescents gained recognition, leading to the expansion of educational opportunities and school attendance.
- Introduction of human growth and development theories: Psychologists Piaget and Erikson introduced theories which placed adolescence as a stage of development as part of achieving adulthood and beyond (Capuzzi & Stauffer, 2016).
- Emergence of teen health programs: The latter half of the twentieth century saw the development of specific programs and initiatives promoting adolescent health issues, including sexual health education and substance abuse prevention.

2.2.3 Twenty-First Century

- Increased access to healthcare: With the expansion of healthcare coverage and programs like Medicaid and the Children's Health Insurance Program (CHIP), more adolescents gained access to essential healthcare services.
- Mental health awareness: There has been a growing awareness of mental health challenges faced by adolescents, leading to increased efforts to address and destigmatize mental health issues.
- Technology and health: The advent of the Internet and mobile technology has facilitated greater access to health information and telemedicine services, benefiting adolescents in remote or underserved areas.
- Growing focus on prevention: There is a stronger emphasis on preventive measures and early intervention strategies, aimed at promoting overall well-being and reducing the burden of chronic diseases in later life.

Despite these improvements, challenges persist in the twenty-first century, including rising rates of obesity, mental health concerns, substance abuse, and health disparities among different populations. Continued efforts are needed to address these challenges and promote the health and well-being of adolescents in the modern era.

2.2.4 The US Timeline

In the USA, the timeline over the past several decades demonstrates structural improvements in health and education.

1960s

- The passage of the Medicaid program in 1965 helps increase access to healthcare services for low-income families, including adolescents.

1970s

- The Title X Family Planning Program is established in 1970, providing access to family planning and reproductive health services for adolescents and low-income individuals.
- The Education for All Handicapped Children Act (now known as the Individuals with Disabilities Education Act) is passed in 1975, ensuring access to education and services for adolescents with disabilities.

1980s

- The Adolescent Health Program is established within the US Centers for Disease Control and Prevention (CDC) to focus on research, policy, and programs related to adolescent health.
- The Drinking Age Act is passed in 1984, raising the legal drinking age to 21 in all states to reduce alcohol-related problems among adolescents.

1990s

- The Personal Responsibility and Work Opportunity Reconciliation Act of 1996 introduces the Temporary Assistance for Needy Families (TANF) program, which includes health coverage for low-income families and adolescents.
- The Children's Health Insurance Program is created in 1997 to provide health coverage for uninsured children and adolescents whose families do not qualify for Medicaid.
- The Mental Health Parity Act was passed in 1996.

2000s

- The Affordable Care Act (ACA) is signed into law in 2010, expanding health insurance coverage and benefits, including preventive services, for adolescents and young adults.
- The US Department of Health and Human Services launches the "Teen Pregnancy Prevention Program" in 2010 to reduce teenage pregnancy rates and promote sexual health education.

2010s

- The opioid epidemic emerges as a major public health concern, impacting adolescents and young adults. Initiatives are launched to address opioid misuse and addiction among this age group.

- Mental health awareness and initiatives to improve access to mental health services become more prominent, given the increasing recognition of mental health challenges faced by adolescents.

2020s

- The COVID-19 pandemic poses significant challenges to adolescent health, affecting education, mental health, and access to healthcare services.
- Efforts to address health disparities and inequities among adolescents gain momentum, focusing on improving health outcomes for marginalized and underserved populations.

Throughout these decades, especially the last two decades, various organizations, healthcare providers, government agencies, and advocacy groups have worked to improve adolescent health through research, policy development, and the implementation of programs and interventions. Adolescent health continues to be an evolving field, with ongoing efforts to enhance the well-being of young people in the USA and globally.

2.3 Adolescent Demographics

According to the 2019 US Census, there are 42 million adolescents living in the USA, comprising 12.8% of the population (U.S. Census Bureau, 2020a). Considering sex assigned at birth, the adolescent numbers are strikingly equivalent (Table 2.1).

While there are slightly more females than males in this age cohort, there is an adolescent wave regarding gender terms who are considering themselves nonbinary. One-half of these adolescents identified themselves as belonging to a racial or ethnic minority.

Racial-ethnic distributions in 2020 are presented in Fig. 2.1 (U.S. Census Bureau, 2020b).

The fact that most adolescents in the USA identify as racial or ethnic minority is important, since typically that subset of the population, especially for African Americans, experiences more health disparities, including health access and insurance.

Table 2.1 Year 2019 distribution of adolescents by age and sex

	Male		Female	
Age in years	Number	Percent	Number	Percent
10–14	10.6 m	0.3	10.2 m	0.3
15–19	10.5 m	0.3	10.2 m	0.3
10–19	21.1 m		20.4 m	

Source: U.S. Census Bureau (2020a)

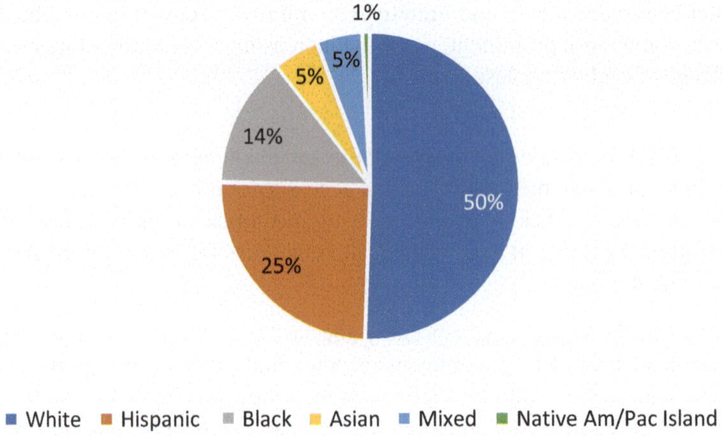

Fig. 2.1 Race/ethnicity of US adolescent population. (U.S. Census Bureau, 2020b)

2.4 Adolescent Development: Psychology and Neurobiology

2.4.1 Theories of Adolescent Psychological Development

Psychological theories of development have typically included behaviors, stages, and periods that were unique to adolescents. Developmental theories describe children at various developmental times and attempt to describe the drivers and constraints of change of shorter and longer time horizons. Most if not all developmental theories sequester changes and constraints into the period of time referred to as adolescence. This time period is differentiated for those before and after. Theories are a critical component of science as they drive questions for more rigorous study. The fact that most developmental theories are imperfect is not a lethal criticism. Many are Eurocentric and are not reflective of non-white cultures.

The history of developmental psychology has been traced to Piaget in the mid twentieth century (Piaget, 1950). His work instituted a shift in psychology that transformed "child psychology" into developmental psychology (Miller, 2023). Although all developmental theories partition the adolescent time frame as separate from children and adults, it has never become a subfield or separate discipline in any of the social professions (e.g., medicine, psychology, psychiatry social work). Whether or not such distinct subfields are good or not misses the point. The point is that adolescence is a distinctly unique phase of development that requires unique knowledge and experience. Its temporal position is roughly the transition from dependence to independence and as such is a social pivot point for the species.

2.4.2 Neurobiology of Adolescent Brain Development

A fundamental concept of neurobiology is that experience shapes the connectivity of specific neural networks. This ability to adapt to environmental influences is termed neural plasticity. This process involves first a growth in neural connections and then a pruning of unused connections (apoptosis). It is not a process of more is better, rather a process where less is more efficient ("better"). Those neural connections used the most get stronger; the others die and get cleaned up. This happens across species and is likely an important aspect of evolutionary fitness (Mishra & Gazzaley, 2016). Further, specific networks become more plastic and change according to timescales tied to other biological changes (Reh et al., 2020). In human development, sensory networks adapt and change first with higher-order emotional and cognitive functions coming later. Adolescent neurodevelopment is driven by these critical periods (CP) that guide the rapid development of neurobiology and cognitive ability during adolescence and their subsequent stability in adulthood (Larsen & Luna, 2018; Uhlhaas et al., 2023).

Studies suggest that during adolescence, their real-time social, emotional, and cognitive experiences alter the structure and function of brain networks subserving these domains of behavior. During this period, the neural networks are more vulnerable and responsive to experience-dependent plasticity. This maturation of neural circuits during adolescence depends, to a large degree, on one's experiences both physical and psychosocial. This occurs through a process of structural and functional adaptation of the nervous system in response to environmental demands, physiological changes, and experiences (Dow-Edwards et al., 2019). Between ages 11 to the early 20s is considered a CP where the development of connections to the prefrontal cortex, hypothalamic-pituitary-adrenal axis (HPA) are notably prolific. These connections subserve the reward system and other functions related to social cognition.

According to this research, the CP in adolescence coincides with the proliferation of neurons specialized for inhibition (parvalbumin-positive (PV) inhibitory neurons; Reh et al., 2020): "These fast-spiking cells generate gamma oscillations associated with critical period plasticity, are sensitive to circadian gene manipulation, emerge at different rates across brain regions, acquire perineuronal nets with age, and may be influenced by epigenetic factors over generations" (Reh et al., 2020, p. 23242).

Higher-order cognitive functions, such as working memory (WM), response inhibition, and performance monitoring, as well as more general cognitive control are central aspects of late brain development, beginning before adolescence and peaking around the age of 18 but continuing into the early 20s. Anatomically, these functions are closely related to the integrity of prefrontal cortical (PFC) circuits that are critical components of reward system function and social cognition (Calabro et al., 2020; Jalbrzikowski et al., 2017; Larsen & Luna, 2018; Park et, al., 2022; Wittmann et al., 2023).

Magnetic resonance imaging (MRI) and functional magnetic resonance imaging (fMRI) studies confirm that adolescence is a period of social brain network neural development (Blakemore, 2012). However, this dramatic neural reorganization also creates a period of vulnerability that increases the possibility for the development of psychopathology. These adolescent brain changes are as significant and striking as changes identified in the first few years of life or even old age. Further, this period of change lasts longer than the period of pubertal change, and adolescent brain maturation extends from 11 to 25 years of age (Lebel & Beaulieu, 2011; Shaw et al., 2008).

During this period, the changes in white and gray matter show increased connectivity between brain regions and increased dopaminergic activity in the prefrontal cortices, striatum, and limbic system and the pathways linking them. The limbic reward systems begin to develop differentially to the top-down control system's heightened responsiveness to incentives, while impulse control is still relatively immature (Casey et al., 2008). Higher-order cognitive functioning, the so-called executive functions, is the last brain region to fully develop in terms of neuronal growth, myelination, and functional connectivity (Institute of Medicine and National Research Council, 2000). While these regions and functions appear to continue developing into adulthood, executive and social brain networks mature during adolescence. Research indicates that adolescents show increased neural reactivity to emotions and rewards, which influences decision-making within social and affective contexts. Thus, it is understandable how adolescence is a sensitive period for social-emotional and self-control learning (Dumontheil, 2016).

In fMRI studies of nonhuman primates, Wittmann and colleagues have characterized the development of different functional reward processes that guide learning. Prior to the onset of puberty, gray matter cortical volumes begin to show growth, particularly in prefrontal areas, and begin a "rewiring" process. The process includes dendrite pruning (underutilized synapses drop out) and increased myelination of axons. Increased myelination both increases the speed of transmission of impulses and thus optimizes information processing. In the end, these processes enhance adolescent neurocircuitry and has been shown to support higher-order cognitive processes of multitasking, problem-solving, and complex thinking (Wittmann et al., 2023).

A distributed network in the human brain supports learning from rewards and making adaptive decisions. This network comprises several regions in lateral and medial prefrontal cortex (PFC), including the lateral and medial orbitofrontal/ventromedial prefrontal cortex, as well as other areas such as the anterior cingulate cortex, the insula cortex, and the amygdala. In concert, they contribute component parts to adaptive behavior such as contingency learning, value comparison, and value representations (Wittmann et al., 2023).

These adaptive behaviors have been operationalized and studied as "local reward learning" and "global reward learning." The former refers to the ability to form contingencies between choice options and outcomes, repeating choices that led to positive outcomes and omitting choices that led to negative outcomes. Global reward learning refers to the reinforcement value of unrelated choices made in close temporal proximity. Noncontingent global reward learning involves forming a representation of a global reward state (GRS), i.e., how much reward was received overall recently independent of the specific choices that caused them (Wittmann et al., 2023). Thus, the integration of specific "lessons" and generalization across "lessons" occur in parallel and become solidified in neural architecture and responsiveness. This reward learning is one of the functions of the basal ganglia, a set of midbrain structures that are involved in voluntary movement as well as initiating higher-order cognitive function (Leisman et al., 2014).

These higher cognitive functions, also called executive functions, include processing signals of emotions, motivations, goal evaluation, risk assessment, planning, and habit formation. Thus, they are key players in certain forms of implicit memory tasks (motor habit learning) and many types of cognitive learning that require repeated trials and are often unconscious and are involved in generated emotional responses. Because of their involvement with reward processing, habit formation, and motivation, the basal ganglia also have an important role in states of well-being and mental illness such as addiction. The basal ganglia are very involved in creating efficiencies within the brain: They recognize and code patterns of stimulus sensation and perception creating templates for fast responses based on previous sequences of learning. Importantly, the basal ganglia's default mode is inhibiting responses so that only "approved," recognized, or reinforcing signals will open the gate to action (Boyes et al., 2022).

These structures change dramatically over the period of adolescence. Recent evidence suggests a link between both a measure of well-being and mental health disorders in young people. Although counterintuitive, the Boyes et al. (2022) study found that reductions in global basal ganglia volume correlated with measures of subjective well-being (positivity and composure) and were linked to regulating stress and negative emotions.

Further, as parental presence varies in phase-like sequences during sensitive periods (e.g., parents going to work, children going to school), there are responses in the recruitment of emotional networks on a moment-to-moment basis (Callaghan & Tottenham, 2016). Their review found that "increasing independence from caregivers cues the termination of the sensitive period for environmental input into emotion network development" (p. 163). This neuro-environmental loop helps the individual to develop stable emotional regulation circuits that are implicated in parental care and the development of amygdala-prefrontal network so critical for emotional functioning.

Clinical data promoting an understanding of peer influences on risky behavior in adolescents provides evidence for the complexity of the roles that peers play in decision-making, a phenomenon different from that in the adult. Imaging studies have revealed that activation of the social network by the presence of peers at times of decision-making is unique in the adolescent. Since normal brain development relies on experiences which alter the functional and structural connections between cells within circuits and networks to ultimately alter behavior, readers can be made aware of the myriad of ways normal developmental processes can be hijacked. The vulnerability of developing adolescent brain places the adolescent at risk for the development of a lifetime of abnormal behaviors and mental disorders (Craiu, 2013). Even though adolescent brain plasticity provides an opportunity to develop talents and lifelong interests, neurotoxic insult, trauma, chronic stress, drug abuse, and sedentary lifestyles may also have negative impacts during this sensitive period of brain maturation (Rosch & Mostofsky, 2019).

Given what has been enumerated based on research of adolescent brain development, three principles stand out:

Principle I Adolescence is the optimum time to provide positive experiences both qualitatively and quantitatively. The adolescent brain is a tumultuous place. The basic wiring has been laid down, but it needs experience to test-drive the system and make it more efficient. What is required is novelty and repetition of (ideally) positive learning experiences. These experiences help to shape adolescent neurobiology, sculpting it as it tries out new possibilities on the road to adulthood.

At the brain level, more is happening so there is more to effect. This means little things have outsized effects (emotional reactivity), while toxic and traumatic experiences can alter function permanently.

In real time, the adolescent brain is vulnerable to social and environmental risks as the frontal lobes prepare for the next 50–70 years. Thus, the crisis of adolescent mental health is not just discomfort or a problem of that age, but it is a problem for the population at large as it portents a crisis in adult functioning in the near future.

Principle II The whole is more than the sum of its parts. As the brain expands its "global reward space," the relative influence of individual choices and reinforcements diminishes, while the accumulation of choice/reinforcement has more influence.

As such, the adolescent and its brain should be considered and treated as a whole. Adolescent learning is far too complex to address with a single domain of expertise, requiring a socio-ecological model that incorporates multiple levels of influence. The consequence of failure in adolescence is long-term dysfunction, potentially lifelong.

Principle III Given these neurobiological changes, it is not surprising that adolescents engage in increased participation of high-risk behaviors. The leading causes of adolescent mortality are accidents, homicide, and suicide. High-risk behaviors include reckless driving, distracted driving, violence, suicidality, substance use and abuse, disordered eating, poor nutrition, and inadequate physical activity.

2.5 The Scope of the Crisis

Adolescence is a transition period and as such is challenging for psychiatric and mental health identification. Many diagnoses of psychopathology are reserved for adults so that a more stable pattern of behavior can be observed or recorded. There is less and less agreement between biological and neurological findings and patient reports of somatic concerns. In the end, a diagnosis of mental illness is in the hands of the clinician.

Several characteristics of adolescent behavior mitigate against diagnostic accuracy with the *Diagnostic and Statistical Manual for Mental Disorders, 5th Ed.* (DSM-5) such that application of the DSM-5 criteria in adolescents can under-identify cases of possible harmful use (American Psychiatric Association, 2013). For instance, differences in how depression presents in adolescents and adults may be consistent with different pathophysiological mechanisms. For adolescents, Rice et al. (2019) found that vegetative/physical disturbances were more common (i.e., loss of energy, changes in weight, appetite and sleep changes). On the other hand, adults reported more anhedonia/loss of interest and concentration difficulties.

This appears to be particularly true for substance use disorder. Symptom definitions need to be clearer and more consistent with the neurodevelopment process and the social aspects that permeate adolescence, which will require further refinement of operational definitions (DeMicheli et al., 2021; Kaminer & Winters, 2015).

Worldwide, the magnitude and prevalence of common mental disorders (CMD) in adolescents has been difficult to track. Silva et al. (2020) completed a meta-analysis of 43 studies looking at common mental disorders in adolescents (10–19 years old). Studies evaluated the CMD prevalence using the standardized General Health Questionnaire (GHQ-12). Global prevalence of CMD in adolescents was 25.0% and 31.0%, using the GHQ cutoff point of 4 and 3, respectively (Bitsko et al., 2022).

Globally, nearly 15% of young people ages 10–19 experience a mental health disorder, accounting for 13% of the global burden of disease in this age group (WHO, 2021a). In 2018–2019, about 15% of adolescents ages 12–17 years had a major depressive episode, 37% had persistent feelings of sadness or hopelessness, and nearly 20% reported that they seriously considered suicide. However, there is now consistent epidemiological evidence that 75% of all mental disorders demonstrate prodromal signs or early indications of mental illness by the age of 25 years (Kessler et al., 2005; Solmi et al., 2022).

Even before the COVID-19 pandemic, worldwide rates of suicide were raising alarms as deaths by suicide became the second leading cause of death in US youth ages 10–24. The blossoming crisis was acknowledged and prompted a joint emergency declaration from the American Academy of Pediatrics, the American Academy of Child and Adolescent Psychiatry, and the Children's Hospital Association: "This worsening crisis in child and adolescent mental health is inextricably tied to the stress brought on by COVID-19 and the ongoing struggle for racial justice and represents an acceleration of trends observed prior to 2020" (American Academy of Pediatrics, 2021).

In 2020, the pooled 1-year prevalence for major depressive disorder (MDD) was 8% (95% CI: 0.05–0.12), and the lifetime prevalence was 19% (95% CI: 0.12–0.26). The point prevalence of elevated depressive symptoms among adolescents between 2001 and 2010 increased from 24% (95% CI: 0.19–0.28) to 37% (95% CI: 0.32–0.42) between 2011 and 2020. (Shorey et al., 2022). Female adolescents were reported to have a higher prevalence of elevated depressive symptoms than male adolescents.

The Racine et al. (2021) meta-analysis of global depression in youth from 2004 to 2020 found similar results in both major depressive episode (MDE) and MDD, which had their highest percentages in 2020, although due to the pandemic, these estimates were probably underreported. The lowest percentage for MDE youth, of 7.9%, occurred in 2006. Likewise, the lowest percentage for MDE with severe impairment occurred during 2006 and 2007 at 5.5%. This represents a significant increase of MDE and MDE with severe impairment for adolescents during this time period (Racine et al., 2021). The data suggested that in the first year of the COVID-19 pandemic, globally one in four youth was experiencing clinically elevated depression symptoms globally (Racine et al., 2021).

The 2021 Mental Health America survey identified the prevalence of youth with a major episode of major depression (MDE) and those with severe MDE, youth with MDE who did not receive mental health services, and those who received some consistent services, all within the past year: 15.08% of youth (aged 12–17) report suffering from at least one major depressive episode (MDE) in the past year. The number of youths experiencing MDE increased by 306,000 (1.24%) from the previous year's dataset (Reinert et al., 2021).

Reinert estimated that 60.3% of youth with major depression do not receive any mental health treatment (Reinert et al., 2021). Youth experiencing MDE continued to go untreated. Even among the states with greatest access for youth, one in three youth is still not receiving the mental health services they need. Nationally, only 27.2% of youth with severe depression receive some consistent treatment (7–25 visits in a year). Consistent treatment was determined if a youth visited a specialty outpatient mental health service, a day treatment facility, mental health clinic, private therapist, or in-home therapist more than seven times in the previous year. Rates of mental health treatment were low for all youth with major depression, and youth of color were significantly less likely to receive depression treatment than white youth. Asian youth were least likely to have seen a health professional or received medication for their depression (8.30%), followed by black or African American youth (9.40%) and Hispanic youth (9.50%) (Substance Use and Mental Health Services Administration, 2020).

2.5.1 Suicide Thoughts and Behaviors Among US Adolescents

Adolescent suicide attempts and deaths have been increasing, especially since the COVID-19 pandemic. In the last quarter of 2020, adolescents were asked if they seriously thought about trying to kill themselves, if they made plans to kill themselves, and if they had tried to kill themselves in the past 12 months. Three million (12%) respondents had serious thoughts of suicide; 1.3 million (5.3%) reported making a suicide plan; and 2.5% or 629,000 (2.5%) attempted suicide in the past year (Substance Abuse and Mental Health Services Administration, 2021, p. 36).

- From 2008 to 2020, the rates of death from suicide among people aged 12 and over increased 16% overall and for youths ages 12–17 increased from 3.7 per 100,000 population to 6.3 per 100,000 population (AHRQ, 2022).

- The rate of suicide death increased by 2% for Hispanic youths from 4.9 per 100,000 population to 5.0 per 100,000 population between 2018 and 2020. The rate for non-Hispanic white youths decreased by 13% from 8.5 per 100,000 population to 7.4 per 100,000 population.

Globally, suicide also ranks as the second leading cause of death for young people aged 15–29 (Campisi et al., 2020; WHO, 2021b). In a study published on adolescent suicide behaviors from 90 countries, one of the key findings was that suicide ideation was dramatically higher for girls than for boys, aged 13–17 (Campisi et al., 2020).

2.5.2 Trauma and Post-traumatic Stress Disorder (PTSD)

Globally, over the past year, over one billion children aged from 2 to 17 years have experienced physical, sexual, or psychological violence or neglect (Maalla M'jid, 2020). Child protection services in the USA reported around 3 million cases of abuse each year involving 5.5 million children with about 30% confirmed, spread across several categories: 65% neglect, 18% physical abuse, 10% sexual abuse, and 7% psychological (mental) abuse.

It is also estimated that three to 10 million children witness family violence each year. Around 40–60% of those cases involve child physical abuse. (Note: It is thought that two-thirds of child abuse cases are not reported.)

Since the Columbine school shooting in 1991, there have been 394 school shootings in the USA which affected over 360,000 students (Washington Post, 2024). Experiences of trauma can cause PTSD and are associated with other psychological disorders, particularly those with more externalizing types of behavior.[1]

PTSD can develop in children and teens even if the traumatic event occurs to someone else. The reaction of others, especially parents, or being physically close to the trauma can add to the severity of response. Thus, any life-threatening event or event that threatens physical harm can cause PTSD. These events may include sexual abuse or violence (Pynoos et al., 1987; see Box 2.1 for list of typical precipitating events).

Box 2.1: Events That Can Precipitate PTSD
- Sexual abuse
- Physical abuse
- Violent crimes
- Environmental disasters
- Floods
- Fires
- Car crashes
- War
- Suicide of someone close
- Seeing violence in the area they live

Indeed, exposure to death or the threat of death is not a necessary precondition. Any event where people are hurt by others, including rape and assault, seems to be more trauma-producing. There also appears to be a dose-response relationship where exposure to more trauma increases the risk of PTSD. Girls are more likely than boys to get PTSD, although the effect of ethnicity on risk is not well-defined (Kessler et al., 2012).

Thus, both the type of event and the intensity of exposure affect risk of PTSD. For example, in one study, the percentage of elementary school children who developed PTSD was directly related to exposure from a fatal sniper attack that occurred in close proximity to the school. Confirming a dose-response relationship, Pynoos et al. documented that moderate to severe PTSD symptoms developed in 77% of the children who directly witnessed the shooting on the playground, while similar moderate to severe symptoms developed in 67% of those in the school building at the time. Only 26% of the children who had gone home for the day had moderate or severe symptoms (Pynoos et al., 1987).

Furthermore, experiencing multiple traumas, such as abuse, community violence, or natural disasters, appears to be common over the course of childhood and adolescence (Finkelhor et al., 2007). Research has demonstrated that poly-victims show more anxiety, depression (Ellonen & Salmi, 2011), less positive school engagement, higher drug usage, and violent behavior than children with experience of a single type of victimization, making this phenomenon a great predictor of traumatic symptoms (Ford et al., 2010). Pires and Almeida's (2023) systematic review provided support for a lifestyles/routine activities framework; that is, youth who engage in activities in unsafe neighborhoods are at increased risk of frequency of victimizations. The increased exposure to trauma in some ethnic minorities may explain why they demonstrate higher symptom loads when they are diagnosed with PTSD (Kessler et al., 2012).

An epidemiological sample of over 10,000 adolescents aged 13–18 estimated that the prevalence of lifetime diagnosis of PTSD would be 5%, with girls 3.5 times greater than boys (8.0% vs. 2.3%) (Merikangas et al., 2010). Overall, according to Kessler et al. (2012), the PTSD 12-month prevalence estimate is 3.9%.

Besides overt exposure, the other risk factors that increase the likelihood of PTSD include female gender, previous trauma exposure, preexisting psychiatric disorders, parental psychopathology, and low social support. Notably, both parental support and lower levels of parental PTSD have been found to predict lower levels of PTSD in children (Williamson et al., 2017). There is less clarity in the findings connecting PTSD with ethnicity and age. While some studies find that minorities report higher levels of PTSD symptoms, researchers have shown that this is due to other factors such as differences in levels of exposure. It is not clear how a child's age at the time of exposure to a traumatic event affects the occurrence or severity of PTSD. While some studies find a relationship, others do not. Differences that do occur may be due to differences in the way PTSD is expressed in children and adolescents of different ages or developmental levels.

Complicating the diagnostic picture, children who experience trauma may also exhibit other problems not necessarily associated with PTSD. For instance, sexually abused children may also struggle with fears, anxiety, depression, anger and hostility, aggression, sexually inappropriate behavior, self-destructive behavior, feelings of isolation and stigma, poor self-esteem, difficulty in trusting others, substance abuse, and sexual maladjustment (Browne & Finkelhor, 1986).

Other co-occurring problems include difficulty with interpersonal relationships, including those with peers and family members; also, adolescents may demonstrate acting out behaviors and lower than expected school performance (American Academy of Child and Adolescent Psychiatry, 2010).

These additional symptoms may rise to the level of diagnosis. Somewhat typical comorbid diagnosed disorders include major depression, substance abuse, anxiety disorders such as separation anxiety, panic disorder, and generalized anxiety disorder and externalizing disorders such as attention-deficit/hyperactivity disorder, oppositional defiant disorder, and conduct disorder (American Academy of Child and Adolescent Psychiatry, 2010).

LeMoult et al. (2020) studied the effect of early life stressors (ELS) and the risk of youth-onset MDD. These included sexual abuse, physical abuse, poverty, physical illness/injury, death of a family member, domestic violence, natural disaster, and emotional abuse. Their meta-analysis revealed that individuals who experienced ELS were more likely to develop MDD before the age of 18 years than were individuals without a history of ELS (odds ratio = 2.50; 95% confidence interval 2.08, 3.00). However, not all ELS were equally contributory, such as poverty.

A study of self-reported symptoms and trauma histories of 94 mixed-sex youth 13–19 years old at four different psychiatric treatment program modalities found that 83% reported experiencing at least one traumatic event. Statistical analysis revealed that more trauma events were associated with externalizing symptoms and PTSD symptoms and severity, after controlling for age, race/ethnicity, gender, and treatment setting. The implication is that those seeking intensive psychiatric care (inpatient psychiatry, outpatient psychiatry, residential substance abuse, and outpatient medical services) have very likely experienced some trauma (American Academy of Child and Adolescent Psychiatry, 2010).

Neurobiologically, adolescent PTSD involves unique neurodevelopmental substrates from adult PTSD, although there is considerable overlap. Fronto-limbic systems development is critical for decision-making and emotional control, which are actively developing in adolescence. While it is not yet known if resilient youth may show less effect, both cross-sectional and longitudinal data suggest abnormal fronto-limbic development compared to typically developing youth (Cisler & Herringa, 2021).

2.5.3 *Anxiety*

Prior to the COVID-19 pandemic, it was estimated that more than 7% of adolescents 13–17 years of age have been diagnosed with anxiety (Ghandour et al., 2019). The National Institute of Mental Health estimated that the prevalence of anxiety disorders in adolescents (13–18 years of age) was 1 in 4 (25%), while the prevalence of severe anxiety was about 1 in 17 (almost 6%) (Walter et al., 2020).

In the first year of the COVID-19 pandemic, it was suggested that globally one in five youth was experiencing clinically elevated anxiety symptoms. These pooled estimates increased over time and are double of those of pre-pandemic estimates. An influx of mental healthcare utilization is expected, and allocation of resources to address child and adolescent mental health concerns is essential (Racine et al., 2021).

Similarly, in a sample of adolescents and young adults living in New York ($n = 451$), Hawes et al. (2022) studied within-person changes in depression and anxiety symptoms from before the pandemic to soon after it first peaked in the spring of 2020. Across participants and independent of age, there were increases in symptoms of generalized anxiety and social anxiety. The effect sizes for change were medium to large (Cohen's -*d*): social anxiety = 0.24, panic symptoms = 0.33, for females overall = 0.38, and generalized anxiety = 0.42.

Prior to COVID, a number of social factors such as pressures to succeed, school shootings, threatening behaviors, climate disruptions, and social media exposure were felt to increase adolescent anxiety. Social media in particular appeared to cause constant comparisons with others that tends to generate feelings of inferiority leading to anxiety. Much of this behavior is modeled or caused by adults that can further cause a sense of loss of control (McCarthy, 2019). COVID-19 likely exacerbated these worrisome trends (Schonfeld, 2024).

2.5.4 Adverse Childhood Experiences (ACEs) and Protective Childhood Experiences (PCEs)

Mental health problems are multiply determined, with both nature (i.e. genetics) and nurture (i.e., social and environmental) playing roles. Adverse childhood experiences, or ACEs, are potentially traumatic events that occur in childhood years (CDC, 2024): Since the ACEs were first published in 1998, it has had an impact in shaping the approach to trauma and how to predict the potential impacts, although it supports a rather dark view of child and adolescent health (Felitti et al., 1998). This negative framing has impacted the approach to research, practice, and discourse about how to move forward to help youth flourish and set the stage for a healthy productive life. Recently the AAP has published a policy brief stating the need to include protective factors that can help to offset the negative impacts of the PCEs (CDC, 2024). This additional focus has coincided with worldwide efforts to focus on health, well-being, and protective factors rather than only the negative outcomes. Boxes 2.2 and 2.3 provide summaries of the ACEs and PCEs.

ACEs are associated with children's physical and mental health. In 2016–2019, among children aged 6–17 years (Merrick et al., 2019)

- Children who were discriminated against based on race or ethnicity had higher percentages of one or more physical health conditions (37.8% versus 27.1%) and one or more mental health conditions (28.9% versus 17.8%) (Hutchins et al., 2022).

Box 2.2: Adverse Childhood Experiences (ACEs)

- Experiencing violence, abuse, or neglect.
- Witnessing violence in the home or community.
- Having a family member attempt or die by suicide.
- Substance use problems.
- Mental health problems.
- Instability due to parental separation.
- Instability due to household members being in jail or prison.

Box 2.3: Protective Childhood Experiences (PCEs)

- Having positive friendships and peer networks.
- Doing well in school.
- Having caring adults outside the family who serve as mentors or role models.
- Safe, stable, and nurturing family relationships, with a consistent, safe, and supported family life.
- Families can meet basic needs of food, shelter, and health services for children and have steady employment.
- Caregivers engage in parental monitoring, supervision, and consistent enforcement of rules.
- Caregivers/adults work through conflicts peacefully.
- Having fun, positive family activities.

- Racial/ethnic discrimination was almost seven times as common among children with three other ACEs compared to those with no other ACEs (Hutchins et al., 2022).

Besides the individual experiences, ACEs are associated with social determinants of health (SDOH). For instance, living in under-resourced or racially segregated neighborhoods can cause toxic stress. Prolonged stress can become toxic and can negatively affect brain development, immune systems, and stress-response systems with consequences for attention, decision-making, and learning (Shonkoff et al., 2012).

Such toxic stress can impact the development of healthy and stable interpersonal relationships and lead to unstable work histories and other socioeconomic difficulties. The effects of historical and ongoing traumas have been shown to pass through generations but can be mediated by stabilized and supportive families (Schofield et al., 2013).

The implication is that experiences and events in a young person's life have long-term implications for health and well-being. A perusal of the protective experiences provides overwhelming support for the protective effect of positive family life.

Indeed, as Callaghan and Tottenham reveal, parental behavior impacts the neurobiology underlying emotional stability (2016).

2.6 Conclusion

Parents do not suddenly relinquish medical decision-making to their children and are a vital part of a process construed within the framework of consent and confidentiality laws. In the transition period from childhood to adulthood, adolescents develop unique healthcare needs and concerns at the very time they are gaining autonomy from their parents. Adolescents progress from being recipients of decisions about their care to gradually becoming active participants in their healthcare and emerge as a primary partner in medical decision-making. Building a strong therapeutic alliance with young people can help them become responsible healthcare decision-makers.

Yet while "healthcare," including mental healthcare, is justifiably viewed as an individual healthcare event, it is part of broader societal need. One's own mental health concerns do not exist in a vacuum. The threats to well-being extend outward to the family, the community, and the wider world. Behavioral, emotional, and cognitive responses are embedded in a culture. And naming the illness does not address the causes. Addressing epidemics requires a longer-range view that rests on prevention and the promotion of healthy, positive behaviors. "Take one and call me in the morning" will not solve any epidemic, including a mental healthcare one.

Given the importance of adolescence as a critical developmental stage with near-term significance for the population's benefit, the current trends of mental health and well-being demonstrate a picture that has been recognized as troubling. It is true that some indicators have shown improvement over the past few decades such as improvements in treatment for severe behavioral disturbance and substance abuse prevalence.

In spite of these challenges, young people are demonstrating creativity, resilience, and commitment when addressing pressing societal issues such as violence, climate change, and inequality. Youth-led social activism related to the environmental movement, such as gun safety and social justice, is a bright spot of purposeful action (Sunrise Movement, n.d.; TEAM ENOUGH, n.d.; Students for Educational Justice, n.d.). And it would be irresponsible to lay blame at the feet of adolescents for the current state of adolescent mental health, who still reside in both developmental and biological phases needing support and leadership. Both professionals and youth have sounded an alarm that much more needs to be done to prepare the next generation of adults who will inherit a troubled planet, including doing more to address their mental health concerns.

Competing Interests *The authors have no conflicts of interest to declare that are relevant to the content of this chapter.*

References

Agency for Healthcare Research and Quality (AHRQ). (2022, October). *2022 National healthcare quality and disparities report*. Pub. No. 22(23)-0030. Retrieved March 25, 2024, from https://www.ahrq.gov/research/findings/nhqrdr/nhqdr22/index.html

American Academy of Child and Adolescent Psychiatry. (n.d.). AACAP History. Retrieved September 5, 2024, from https://www.aacap.org/AACAP/About_AACAP/AACAP_History.aspx

American Academy of Child and Adolescent Psychiatry. (2010). Practice parameters for the assessment and treatment of children and adolescents with posttraumatic stress disorder. *Journal of the American Academy of Child and Adolescent Psychiatry, 49*, 414–430.

American Academy of Pediatrics. (2021). *Declaration of a national emergency in child and adolescent mental health*. Retrieved 25 Jan 2023, from https://www.aap.org/en/advocacy/child-and-adolescent-healthy-mental-development/aap-aacap-cha-declaration-of-a-national-emergency-in-child-and-adolescent-mental-health/

American Psychiatric Association. (2013). *Diagnostic and statistical manual of mental disorders* (5th ed.). American Psychiatric Publishing.

Barthel, R. P. (2007). The American Academy of Child and Adolescent Psychiatry. *Academic Psychiatry, 31*(2), 119–121.

Bitsko, R. H., Claussen, A. H., Lichtstein, J., Black, L. J., Jones, S. E., Danielson, M. D., Hoenig, J. M., Davis Jack, S. P., Brody, D. J., Gyawali, S., Maenner, M. J., Warner, M., Holland, K. M., Perou, R., Crosby, A. E., Blumberg, S. J., Avenevoli, S., Kaminski, J. W., & Ghandour, R. M. (2022, February 25). Mental health surveillance among children—United States, 2013–2019. *MMWR Supplements, 71*(2), 1–42. Retrieved October 4, 2022, from https://www.cdc.gov/mmwr/volumes/71/su/su7102a1.htm

Blakemore, S. (2012). Imaging brain development: The adolescent brain. *NeuroImage, 61*, 397–406.

Boyes, A., McLoughlin, L. T., Anderson, H., Schwenn, P., Shan, Z., Gatt, J. M., Lagopoulos, J., & Hermens, D. F. (2022). Basal ganglia correlates of wellbeing in early adolescence. *Brain Research, 1774*, 147710. https://doi.org/10.1016/j.brainres.2021.147710

Browne, A., & Finkelhor, D. (1986). Impact of child sexual abuse: A review of the research. *Psychological Bulletin, 99*, 66–77.

Calabro, F. J., Murty, V. P., Jalbrzikowski, M., Tervo-Clemmens, B., & Luna, B. (2020). Development of hippocampal-prefrontal cortex interactions through adolescence. *Cerebral Cortex, 30*, 1548–1558.

Callaghan, B., & Tottenham, M. (2016). *Neuropsychopharmacology Reviews, 41*, 163–176. https://doi.org/10.1038/npp.2015.204; published online 2 September 2015.

Campisi, S. C., Carducci, B., Akseer, N., et al. (2020). Suicidal behaviours among adolescents from 90 countries: A pooled analysis of the global school-based student health survey. *BMC Public Health, 20*(1), 1102. https://doi.org/10.1186/s12889-020-09209-z

Capuzzi, D., & Stauffer, M. D. (Eds.). (2016). *Human growth and development across the lifespan: Applications for counselors*. Wiley. https://doi.org/10.1002/9781394258925

Casey, B. J., Getz, S., & Galavan, A. (2008). The adolescent brain. *Developmental Review, 28*(1), 62–77.

Centers for Disease Control and Prevention (CDC). (2024). *Risk and protective factors*. Retrieved March 7, 2024, https://www.cdc.gov/aces/about/?CDC_AAref_Val=https://www.cdc.gov/violenceprevention/aces/fastfact.html

Cisler, J. M., & Herringa, R. J. (2021). Posttraumatic stress disorder and the developing adolescent brain. *Biological Psychiatry, 89*(2), 144–151. https://doi.org/10.1016/j.biopsych.2020.06.001

Clark, H., Ghebreyesus, T. A., Albrectsen, A., Alcocer, J., Alden, E., Azoulay, A., et al. (2021). Uniting for adolescents in covid-19 and beyond. *BMJ, 372*, n7190. https://doi.org/10.1136/bmj.n719

Craiu, D. (2013). What is special about the adolescent (JME) brain? *Epilepsy & Behavior, 28*(Suppl 1), S45–S51. https://doi.org/10.1016/j.yebeh.2012.12.008

DeMicheli, D., Andrade, A. L. M., & Galduróz, J. C. (2021). Limitations of DSM-5 diagnostic criteria for substance use disorder in adolescents: What have we learned after using these criteria for several years? *Brazilian Journal of Psychiatry, 43*(4), 349–350. https://doi.org/10.1590/1516-4446-2020-1151

Dow-Edwards, D., MacMaster, F. P., Peterson, B. S., Niesink, R., Andersen, S., & Braams, B. R. (2019, November–December). Experience during adolescence shapes brain development: From synapses and networks to normal and pathological behavior. *Neurotoxicology and Teratology, 76*, 106834. https://doi.org/10.1016/j.ntt.2019.106834

Dumontheil, I. (2016). Adolescent brain development. *Current Opinion in Behavioral Sciences, 10*, 39–44. https://doi.org/10.1016/j.cobeha.2016.04.012

Ellonen, N., & Salmi, V. (2011). Poly-victimization as a life condition: Correlates of poly-victimization among Finnish children. *Journal of Scandinavian Studies in Criminology and Crime Prevention, 12*(1), 20–44. https://doi.org/10.1080/14043858.2011.561621

Felitti, V. J., Anda, R. F., Nordenberg, D., Williamson, D. F., Spitz, A. M., Edwards, V., Koss, M. P., & Marks, J. S. (1998). Relationship of childhood abuse and household dysfunction to many of the leading causes of death in adults. The adverse childhood experiences (ACE) study. *American Journal of Preventive Medicine, 14*(4), 245–258. https://doi.org/10.1016/s0749-3797(98)00017-8

Finkelhor, D., Ormrod, R. K., & Turner, H. A. (2007). Poly-victimization: A neglected component in child victimization. *Child Abuse & Neglect: The International Journal, 31*, 7–26. https://doi.org/10.1016/j.chiabu.2006.06.008

Ford, J. D., Elhai, J. D., Connor, D. F., & Frueh, B. C. (2010). Poly-victimization and risk of posttraumatic, depressive, and substance use disorders and involvement in delinquency in a national sample of adolescents. *Journal of Adolescent Health, 46*(6), 545–552. https://doi.org/10.1016/j.jadohealth.2009.11.212

Ghandour, R. M., Sherman, L. J., Vladutiu, C. J., et al. (2019). Prevalence and treatment of depression, anxiety, and conduct problems in US children. *Journal of Pediatrics, 206*, 256–267.e3.

Hawes, M. T., Szenczy, A. K., Klein, D. N., Hajcak, G., & Nelson, B. D. (2022). Increases in depression and anxiety symptoms in adolescents and young adults during the COVID-19 pandemic. *Psychological Medicine, 52*(14), 3222–3230. https://doi.org/10.1017/S0033291720005358

Hutchins, H. J., Barry, C. M., Valentine, V., Bacon, S., Njai, R., Claussen, A. H., Ghandour, R. M., Lebrun-Harris, L. A., Perkins, K., & Robinson, L. R. (2022). Perceived racial/ethnic discrimination, physical and mental health conditions in childhood, and the relative role of other adverse experiences. *Adversity and Resilience Science*. Published online May 23, 2022.

Institute of Medicine and National Research Council. (2000). *From neurons to neighborhoods: The science of early childhood development*. The National Academies Press. https://doi.org/10.17226/9824

Jalbrzikowski, M., Larsen, B., Hallquist, M. N., Foran, W., Calabro, F., & Luna, B. (2017). Development of white matter microstructure and intrinsic functional connectivity between the amygdala and ventromedial prefrontal cortex: Associations with anxiety and depression. *Biological Psychiatry, 82*, 511–521.

Kaminer, Y., & Winters, K. C. (2015). DSM-5 criteria for youth substance use disorders: Lost in translation? *Journal of the American Academy of Child and Adolescent Psychiatry, 54*(5), 350–351. https://doi.org/10.1016/j.jaac.2015.01.016

Kessler, R. C., Berglund, P., Demler, O., Jin, R., Merikangas, K. R., & Walters, E. E. (2005). Lifetime prevalence and age-of-onset distributions of DSM-IV disorders in the National Comorbidity Survey Replication. *Archives of General Psychiatry, 62*, 593–602.

Kessler, R. C., Avenevoli, S., Costello, E. J., Georgiades, K., Green, J. G., Gruber, M. J., He, J. P., Koretz, D., McLaughlin, K. A., Petukhova, M., Sampson, N. A., Zaslavsky, A. M., & Merikangas, K. R. (2012, April). Prevalence, persistence, and sociodemographic correlates of

DSM-IV disorders in the National Comorbidity Survey Replication Adolescent Supplement. *Archives of General Psychiatry, 69*(4), 372–380.

Larsen, B., & Luna, B. (2018). Adolescence as a neurobiological critical period for the development of higher-order cognition. *Neuroscience and Biobehavioral Reviews, 94*, 179–195.

Lebel, C., & Beaulieu, C. (2011). Longitudinal development of human brain wiring continues from childhood into adulthood. *The Journal of Neuroscience, 31*, 10937–10947.

Lee, L., Upadhya, K. K., Matson, P. A., Adger, H., & Trent, M. E. (2016). The status of adolescent medicine: Building a global adolescent workforce. *International Journal of Adolescent Medicine and Health, 28*(3), 233–243. https://doi.org/10.1515/ijamh-2016-5003. PMID: 26167974; PMCID: PMC5039240.

Leisman, G., Braun-Benjamin, O., & Melillo, R. (2014). Cognitive-motor interactions of the basal ganglia in development. *Frontiers in Systems Neuroscience, 8*, 1–18.

LeMoult, J., Humphreys, K. L., Tracy, A., Hoffmeister, J. A., Ip, E., & Gotlib, I. H. (2020). Meta-analysis: Exposure to early life stress and risk for depression in childhood and adolescence. *Journal of the American Academy of Child and Adolescent Psychiatry, 59*(7), 842–855. https://doi.org/10.1016/j.jaac.2019.10.011

Maalla M'jid, N. (2020). Hidden scars: The impact of violence and the COVID-19 pandemic on children's mental health. *Child and Adolescent Psychiatry and Mental Health, 14*, 33. https://doi.org/10.1186/s13034-020-00340-8

McCarthy, C. (2019). Anxiety in teens is rising. What's going on? *Healthy Kids*. American Academy of Pediatrics. https://www.healthychildren.org/English/health-issues/conditions/emotional-problems/Pages/Anxiety-Disorders.aspx

Merikangas, K. R., He, J. P., Burstein, M., Swanson, S. A., Avenevoli, S., Cui, L., Benjet, C., Georgiades, K., & Swendsen, J. (2010, October). Lifetime prevalence of mental disorders in U.S. adolescents: Results from the National Comorbidity Survey Replication—Adolescent Supplement (NCS-A). *Journal of the American Academy of Child and Adolescent Psychiatry, 49*(10), 980–989.

Merrick, M. T., Ford, D. C., Ports, K. A., Guinn, A. N., et al. (2019). Vital signs: Estimated proportion of adult health problems attributable to adverse childhood experiences and implications for prevention—25 states, 2015–2017. *MMWR. Morbidity and Mortality Weekly Report, 68*, 999–1005. https://doi.org/10.15585/mmwr.mm6844e1

Miller, P. (2023). Developmental theories: Past, present, and future. *Developmental Review, 66*, 1–13. https://doi.org/10.1016/j.dr.2022.101049

Mishra, J., & Gazzaley, A. (2016). Cross-species approaches to cognitive neuroplasticity research. *NeuroImage, 131*, 4–12. https://doi.org/10.1016/j.neuroimage.2015.09.002

O'Neill, A. (n.d.). *Life expectancy (from birth) in the United States, from 1860 to 2020*. Statista. Retrieved March 7, 2024, from https://www.statista.com/statistics/1040079/life-expectancy-united-states-all-time/

Park, B. Y., Paquola, C., Bethlehem, R., Benkarim, O., Mišić, B., & Neuroscience in Psychiatry Network (NSPN) Consortium. (2022). Adolescent development of multiscale structural wiring and functional interactions in the human connectome. *Proceedings of the National Academy of Sciences of the United States of America, 119*, e2116673119.

Piaget, J. (1950). *The psychology of intelligence*. Harcourt, Brace.

Pires, A. R., & Almeida, T. C. (2023). Risk factors of poly-victimization and the impact on delinquency in youth: A systematic review. *Crime & Delinquency*. https://doi.org/10.1177/00111287221148656

Protecting Youth Mental Health: The U.S. Surgeon General's Advisory. (2021). U.S. Government Printing Office. Retrieved February 29. 2024, from https://www.hhs.gov/sites/default/files/surgeon-general-youth-mental-health-advisory.pdf

Pynoos, R. S., Frederick, C., Nader, K., Arroyo, W., Steinberg, A., Eth, S., Nunez, F., & Fairbanks, L. (1987, December). Life threat and posttraumatic stress in school-age children. *Archives of General Psychiatry, 44*(12), 1057–1063. https://doi.org/10.1001/archpsyc.1987.01800240031005

Racine, N., McArthur, B. A., Cooke, J. E., Eirich, R., Zhu, J., & Madigan, S. (2021, November 1). Global prevalence of depressive and anxiety symptoms in children and adolescents during COVID-19: A meta-analysis. *JAMA Pediatrics, 175*(11), 1142–1150. https://doi.org/10.1001/jamapediatrics.2021.2482

Reh, R. K., Dias, B. G., Nelson, C. A., 3rd, Kaufer, D., Werker, J. F., Kolb, B., Levine, J. D., & Hensch, T. K. (2020). Critical period regulation across multiple timescales. *Proceedings of the National Academy of Sciences of the United States of America, 117*(38), 23242–23251. https://doi.org/10.1073/pnas.1820836117

Reinert, M., Fritze, D., & Nguyen, T. (2021, October). *The state of mental health in America 2022.* Mental Health America.

Rice, F., Riglin, L., Lomax, T., Souter, E., Potter, R., Smith, D. J., Thapar, A. K., & Thapar, A. (2019). Adolescent and adult differences in major depression symptom profiles. *Journal of Affective Disorders, 15*(243), 175–181. https://doi.org/10.1016/j.jad.2018.09.015

Rosch, K. S., & Mostofsky, S. (2019). Development of the frontal lobe. *Handbook of Clinical Neurology, 163*, 351–367. https://doi.org/10.1016/B978-0-12-804281-6.00019-

Schofield, T. J., Lee, R. D., & Merrick, M. T. (2013). Safe, stable, nurturing relationships as a moderator of intergenerational continuity of child maltreatment: A meta-analysis. *The Journal of Adolescent Health, 53*(4 Suppl), S32–S38. https://doi.org/10.1016/j.jadohealth.2013.05.004

Schonfeld, D. (2024). *How to talk with kids about tragedies & other traumatic news events.* American Academy of Pediatrics.

Shaw, P., Kabani, N. J., Lerch, J. P., Eckstrand, K., Lenroot, R., Gogtay, N., et al. (2008). Neurodevelopmental trajectories of the human cerebral cortex. *The Journal of Neuroscience, 28*, 3586–3594.

Shonkoff, J. P., Garner, A. S., & Committee on Psychosocial Aspects of Child and Family Health, Committee on Early Childhood, Adoption, and Dependent Care, & Section on Developmental and Behavioral Pediatrics. (2012). The lifelong effects of early childhood adversity and toxic stress. *Pediatrics, 129*(1), e232–e246. https://doi.org/10.1542/peds.2011-2663

Shorey, S., Ng, E. D., & Wong, C. H. J. (2022). Global prevalence of depression and elevated depressive symptoms among adolescents: A systematic review and meta-analysis. *The British Journal of Clinical Psychology, 61*(2), 287–305. https://doi.org/10.1111/bjc.12333. Epub 2021 Sep 26. PMID: 34569066.

Silva, S. A., Silva, S. U., Ronca, D. B., Gonçalves, V. S. S., Dutra, E. S., & Carvalho, K. M. B. (2020 April 23). Common mental disorders prevalence in adolescents: A systematic review and meta-analyses. *PLoS One, 15*(4), e0232007. https://doi.org/10.1371/journal.pone.0232007

Solmi, M., Radua, J., Olivola, M., Croce, E., Soardo, L., Salazar de Pablo, G., et al. (2022). Age at onset of mental disorders worldwide: Large-scale meta-analysis of 192 epidemiological studies. *Molecular Psychiatry, 27*, 281–295.

Students for Educational Justice. (n.d.). *Youth led organizing and training*. https://students4edjustice.org/our-work/youth-led-organizing-and-training/

Substance Abuse and Mental Health Services Administration. (2021). *Key substance use and mental health indicators in the United States: Results from the 2020 National Survey on Drug Use and Health* (HHS Publication No. PEP21-07-01-003, NSDUH Series H-56). Center for Behavioral Health Statistics and Quality, Substance Abuse and Mental Health Services Administration. Retrieved December 20, 2023, from https://www.samhsa.gov/data/

Substance Use and Mental Health Services Administration. (2020). *National survey on drug use and health (NSDUH).* U.S. Department of Health and Human Services, Substance Abuse and Mental Health Services Administration (SAMHSA), Center for Behavioral Health Statistics and Quality. (2018–2019). National Survey on Drug Use and Health 2018–2019. Retrieved December 20, 2023, from https://rdas.samhsa.gov

Sunrise Movement. (n.d.). Retrieved January 20, 2024, from https://www.sunrisemovement.org/

TEAM ENOUGH. (n.d.). *TEAM ENOUGH: We are saying enough.* [Brady organization]. https://www.teamenough.org/

U.S. Census Bureau. (2020a). *Current population survey, annual social and economic supplement, 2019.* U.S. Census Bureau, Population Division. Retrieved October 31, 2022, from https://www2.census.gov/programs-surveys/demo/tables/age-and-sex/2019/age-sex-composition/2019gender_table1.xlsx

U.S. Census Bureau. (2020b). *Annual estimates of the resident population by sex, age, race, and Hispanic origin for the United States: April 1, 2010 to July 1, 2019* (NC-EST2019-ASR6H). Retrieved October 31, 2022, from https://www.census.gov/newsroom/press-kits/2020/population-estimates-detailed.html

Uhlhaas, P. J., Davey, C. G., Mehta, U. M., Shah, J., Torous, J., Allen, N. B., et al. (2023). Towards a youth mental health paradigm: A perspective and roadmap. *Molecular Psychiatry, 28*(8), 3171–3181. https://doi.org/10.1038/s41380-023-02202-z

Walter, H. J., Bukstein, O. G., Abright, A. R., et al. (2020). Clinical practice guideline for the assessment and treatment of children and adolescents with anxiety disorders. *Journal of the American Academy of Child and Adolescent Psychiatry, 59*(10), 1107–1124. https://doi.org/10.1016/j.jaac.2020.05.005

Washington Post. (2024). Retrieved February 10, 2024, from https://www.washingtonpost.com/education/interactive/school-shootings-database/

Williamson, V., Creswell, C., Fearon, P., Hiller, R. M., Walker, J., & Halligan, S. L. (2017). The role of parenting behaviors in childhood post-traumatic stress disorder: A meta-analytic review. *Clinical Psychology Review, 53*, 1–13. https://doi.org/10.1016/j.cpr.2017.01.005

Wittmann, M. K., Scheuplein, M., Gibbons, S. G., & Noonan, M. P. (2023). Local and global reward learning in the lateral frontal cortex show differential development during human adolescence. *PLoS Biology, 21*(3), e3002010. https://doi.org/10.1371/journal.pbio.3002010

World Health Organization. (2002). *Adolescent friendly health services: An agenda for change.* Retrieved January 20, 2024, from https://iris.who.int/bitstream/handle/10665/67923/WHO_FCH_CAH_02.14.pdf.

World Health Organization. (2021a, November). *Mental health of adolescents.* Retrieved October 4, 2022, from https://www.who.int/news-room/fact-sheets/detail/adolescent-mental-health

World Health Organization. (2021b). *Suicide worldwide in 2019: Global health estimates.* WHO.

Chapter 3
School Mental Health Milestones Since the Late Twentieth Century

Donna Lord Black

3.1 Public Education, School Health, and Adolescent Mental Health

Social scientists have long recognized the role of public education in creating, establishing, and enhancing a society's well-being. The interdependent relationship between societies and their public education systems has been well-documented in the research (Francois, 2015), and it has been shown that schools play an integral role in developing healthy, robust, and productive societies. An investment in a society's public education system provides the foundation for the human capital necessary for a healthy economy that offers healthy dividends. Therefore, an investment in public education is an investment in a society's future (Aspen Institute, n.d.).

Whenever mental health problems exist in a society, they threaten to undermine the overall health and well-being of the society. This threat is not restrained by boundaries but extends to all people in the society regardless of age, race, gender, religion, ethnicity, or culture. Schools are not exempted from this threat but are far more likely to experience its impact because school and related activities are where young people spend a large amount of their time. Mental health problems in schools when gone unchecked and untreated not only can disrupt the learning environment but also can strain the limited resources of a school and place added burdens on its staff and students (World Health Organization, 2023).

Since school is where most students spend a large amount of their time and where they encounter "real-life" situations and challenges, it is perhaps the most

D. L. Black (✉)
Independent Educational Consultant, Frisco, TX, USA

Social-Emotional Learning Alliance for Texas (SEL4TX.org), Frisco, TX, USA

Academy for Social-Emotional Learning in Schools, Rutgers University, Rutgers, NJ, USA
e-mail: dblack@sel4tx.org

P. G. Bray, A. Maerlender (eds.), *Adolescent Public Mental Health*,
https://doi.org/10.1007/978-3-031-68294-0_3

ecologically effective environment for delivering these services (Weist et al., 2023), but mental health resources in schools are in short supply. This shortage is not confined to schools. Data from the US Health Resources and Services Administration reports that mental health has been designated as a Health Professional Shortage Area (HPSA) in the USA, and the total number of practitioners needed to fill this shortage, whether in schools or in communities, surpasses 6000 (Health Resources and Services Administration, 2024).

With resources for mental health services in short supply, schools and communities are challenged to provide mental health supports and interventions for adolescents. According to the US Department of Education (2023), more than one in three high school students reported experiencing poor mental health during the height of the COVID-19 pandemic. Despite this need, only 37.6% of all public schools in the USA were able to provide mental health treatment to its students during the 2021–2022 school year (Burr et al., 2024). According to the National Association of School Psychologists (NASP), it is estimated that schools have a current ratio of 1 school psychologist for every 1127 students (1:1127). The recommended ratio, however, is 1 school psychologist for every 500 students (1:500). The NASP also estimates that this ratio varies significantly among all states and some states are approaching a ratio of 1 school psychologist for every 5000 students (1:5000). Furthermore, the NASP also projects it will take an additional 60,000 school psychologists to adequately staff schools in the USA, which could take between 20 and 25 years (National Association of School Psychologists, n.d.). Among other school mental health service providers, the number of school counselors is also in short supply. In a survey of school counseling directors, 68% reported there were not enough school counselors to fill positions in their states, and 55% reported there were not enough to fill positions in their districts (American School Counselor Association, 2023).

Even when schools are staffed with enough secondary school counselors, their roles and responsibilities vary greatly across schools and districts. Most secondary school counselors do not provide direct mental health services in schools because other equally important responsibilities demand most of their time. These include helping students with their academic schedules, assisting them with college applications, and helping them with transitioning to life after high school (American School Counselor Association, 2019). As a result, direct mental health services are not likely to be prioritized unless there is a crisis.

While physical and mental health treatment are both of critical importance and deserving of our best resources and supports, historically there has been greater neglect in the funding of mental health needs than in the funding of physical health needs. To further complicate the problem, efforts to help schools address and prevent mental health problems are often underfunded and of a low priority in the USA and many developed societies. Relatedly, this underfunding of mental health treatment has become a global concern despite mandates to create parity between mental health and physical health. According to Mahomed (2020), mental health treatment remains a neglected priority of policymakers and funders, and this constitutes a glaring neglect of human rights just as it would if physical health needs were ignored. As a result of this underfunding, school resources for mental health intervention are extremely limited, and efforts are often more reactive than preventive.

Mental health problems among young people are often precipitated and/or exacerbated by certain environmental factors, among which poverty, abuse, neglect, substance use, and exposure to violence are the most salient. These precipitating/exacerbating factors not only create barriers to learning and achievement, but they also lead to inequitable and poor outcomes for these students and for the school systems that serve them (Fig. 3.1). The COVID-19 pandemic has worsened the impact of these barriers on student mental health and has highlighted the fact that much of the mental healthcare in the USA occurs in a silo, disconnected from the care of other health conditions (Scott et al., 2023). The barriers to learning and achievement and the concurrent mental health crisis in schools (American Academy of Child and Adolescent Psychiatry, American Academy of Pediatrics, and Children's Hospital Association, 2021) cannot be solved through academic support alone but must be addressed through early intervention and prevention efforts and through mental health literacy (Adelman & Taylor, 2005). A coordinated and collaborative process guided by a multitiered problem-solving framework is one approach that has been proven effective, and schools can, and should, play a fundamental role in this process.

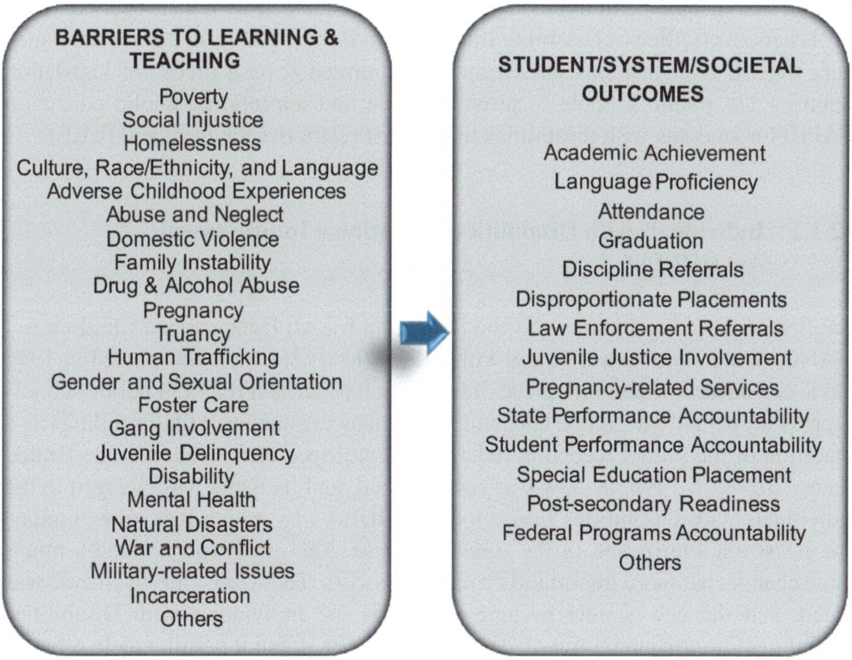

Fig. 3.1 Making connections Barriers to learning that create inequitable outcomes for schools, systems, and society. (Source: Black (2022a). Adapted and reprinted with permission of the publisher)

3.2 Tiered Prevention Frameworks

3.2.1 Historical Context

"History cannot give us a program for the future, but it can give us a fuller understanding of ourselves, and of our common humanity, so that we can better face the future" (Warren, 1961).

3.2.1.1 Civil Rights for Students with Disabilities

Prior to 1975, regular educational practices in the USA excluded children with certain types of disabilities from attending and participating in school. In the early 1970s, more than 3.5 million children with disabilities such as emotional disturbance, mental retardation, blindness, and deafness were simply being warehoused in segregated facilities or state institutions where they had no access to public education and received little or no effective instruction (Individuals with Disabilities Education Act, 2024). In 1973, civil rights advocates and parents of children with disabilities lobbied Congress to pass the first federal legislation to address civil rights for people with disabilities. Section 504 of the Rehabilitation Act of 1973 ensured that disabled children had the right to be educated with their peers in regular classrooms (Office of Disability Employment Policy, 2023). In the decades since then, the US Congress has passed and reauthorized several pieces of legislation requiring US public schools to provide a free and appropriate public education (FAPE) for students with disabilities in the least restrictive environment (LRE).

3.2.1.2 Individuals with Disabilities Educational Improvement Act (IDEIA)

The first of these legislations was the Education for All Handicapped Children Act (EAHCA), also known as EHA or Public Law 94–142, which was passed in 1975 and is considered a landmark piece of legislation because it required public schools to provide specially designed educational services to students with disabilities as a condition of the school receiving federal funding (Special Education in the United States, 2024). In 1990, the law was reauthorized, and its name was changed to the Individuals with Disabilities Education Act (IDEA), by which it is known today. The latest reauthorization of the statute came in 2004, and with it came a minor name change, but more importantly a named process. The word "improvement" was added, and the new statute became known as the Individuals with Disabilities Educational Improvement Act of 2004, or IDEIA 2004, but it is still widely referred to as IDEA (U.S. Department of Education, n.d.-a). The process added in 2004, response to intervention (RTI), was a multitiered approach through which schools could document student intervention efforts and, depending on the state, was used to determine the need for referral for special services (Berkeley et al., 2020).

With each reauthorization of the statute, definitions were provided for each disability category under which students could be considered eligible for services. The current 2004 version includes definitions for 13 disability categories, and of these 13 categories, the definition of emotional disturbance remains the same as it was in the original statute that was passed in 1975 (Individuals with Disabilities Education Act, n.d.). This dated definition of emotional disturbance lacks research support, adds complexity and confusion regarding what constitutes an emotional disturbance, and promotes a "wait-and-fail" approach to identification (Landrum & Kauffman, n.d.).

3.2.1.3 No Child Left Behind Act (NCLB)

Previous efforts to ensure access to public education services for students with disabilities were later aligned with other pieces of legislation which regulated education services for "all" students. Specifically, the reauthorization of IDEIA 2004 was a significant attempt to align it with the Elementary and Secondary Education Act (ESEA) which had been reauthorized and renamed (No Child Left Behind Act (NCLB), 2001). This alignment of IDEA with NCLB was significant in that it laid the groundwork for subsequent pieces of legislation that would impact the future of public education for "all" students (Individuals with Disabilities Education Act, n.d.).

A notable event prompting changes in the educational landscape of the USA was the publication of a volume of papers which examined the past, present, and future of special education (Finn et al., 2001). Those findings acknowledged that while IDEA had been successful in providing increased access to educational opportunities for students with disabilities, it also had resulted in several unintended negative outcomes. Among these was a burgeoning growth in the identification and eligibility of students with specific learning disabilities (SLDs). The number of students identified as having an SLD had grown by more than 233% since 1976, while the numbers of students identified in the other disability categories had grown only by 13% during the same time frame. Among these other disability categories, the number of students identified as having the disability of emotional disturbance had decreased, while classroom behavioral concerns and discipline issues had risen. Furthermore, outcome studies for students identified with an emotional disturbance suggested these students had fared worse than students from all other categories of disabilities (Newman et al., 2009).

The passage of NCLB, along with the volume of papers published by Finn and colleagues, led to an increased concern for accountability in public education and an increased focus on educational reform efforts. In 2002, the President's Commission on Excellence in Special Education was formed for the purpose of examining the state of special education in the USA (Exec. Order No. 13227, 2001). Upon completion of its work, the commission published a report containing recommendations for special education services and how they could be improved. First, it recommended that schools start focusing on results and not on processes. Next, it recommended that schools embrace a model of prevention, not a model of failure. Lastly, it recommended that children with disabilities be considered as general education students first and be provided access to the same curriculum and high-quality instruction as their nondisabled peers (President's Commission on Excellence in Special Education, 2002).

3.2.1.4 Every Student Succeeds Act (ESSA)

For the next decade and more, increased accountability became the driving force behind efforts in the USA to reform and improve student and system outcomes in public education. The NCLB Act had been armed with many prescriptive requirements for schools, and these accountability directives eventually became unworkable for schools. In recognition of this, Congress reauthorized the Act in December 2015 and replaced it with the Every Student Succeeds Act (ESSA). With this reauthorization, the federal government's role in education became narrower, and states were given greater control in designing their own educational programs and accountability systems (U.S. Department of Education, n.d.-b). The Act provided states with more flexibility regarding some of the specific requirements contained in NCLB, and, in exchange, they were to focus on preparing students for success in college and careers. In addition, each state was required to develop a rigorous plan to help close the achievement gap for traditionally underserved populations of students. The Act also stipulated that state plans should contain efforts to increase equity and ensure access to high-quality instruction for all students (U.S. Department of Education, 2017).

3.2.1.5 Flexibility in the Use of Federal Funds and a Focus on Prevention

One of the significant changes that came from ESSA was that schools were given additional flexibility in how to spend federal funds. Prior to ESSA, schools were required to spend their federal funds on the program the grant was intended to support, but the new requirements in ESSA allowed multiple grant funds to be woven, or "braided," together to support schoolwide efforts for student improvement. Coordinated spending of these funds was allowed, so long as the activities for which the funds were being used were permitted under the grant program. In such cases, schools were required to maintain documentation on how the federal funds were being spent for each source of funding. Schools also could combine or "blend" certain funds to support certain circumstances (Office of Disability Employment Policy, n.d.). Under ESSA, braiding and blending of federal funds allowed schools to coordinate their resources and avoid duplication of services.

Another significant change resulting from ESSA was rethinking the response to intervention (RTI) model that had been introduced with NCLB for addressing struggling students. ESSA moved schools toward a more prevention-focused framework called multitiered system of supports (MTSS). Using MTSS, schools could affect systemic change by intentionally integrating programs, resources, and supports. Additionally, schools could align their efforts to address the needs of the whole child, including their academic, social, emotional, and behavioral needs. While ESSA encouraged schools to use braiding of their funds to support an MTSS framework, they were not mandated to do so.

3.2.1.6 COVID-19 Pandemic Brings Challenges for Public Education

Despite their flexibility in how they use their ESSA funds, schools have continued to struggle with meeting the social, emotional, and behavioral needs of their students. In 2020, the COVID-19 pandemic drove these challenges into unprecedented territory (United Nations, 2020). Beginning in late February 2020, most schools in the USA began closing and providing instruction to students over the Internet and did not begin to reopen until August 2020. The prolonged isolation and social distancing, while it impacted all ages, was most debilitating for children, adolescents, and young adults. As the pandemic progressed, concerns for their social and emotional well-being widened, and it became increasingly clear that the afflictions brought on by the pandemic had extended far beyond students' academic development. Furthermore, these afflictions were far greater for children of lower socioeconomic status. Consequently, as schools began to reopen in August 2020, academic achievement and social-emotional development became a top priority. While data showed significant learning losses had occurred for most students, the racial achievement gap that already existed prior to the pandemic had widened further (Goldhaber et al., 2022). Although the long-term implications of the pandemic for young peoples' social-emotional development have not yet been fully determined (National Academies of Sciences, Engineering, & Medicine, 2023), studies have shown clearly that mental health problems have risen (Araújo et al., 2021).

3.2.1.7 Elementary and Secondary School Emergency Relief (ESSER)

To assist schools in reopening after the pandemic, the US Congress passed three relief packages known as the Elementary and Secondary School Emergency Relief (ESSER) funds. These time-limited funds were intended to help schools prevent, prepare for, and respond to the pandemic's impact on the academic, social, emotional, and mental health needs of their students. For many schools, the funds brought welcomed relief and support for their academic improvement efforts, but when it came to addressing students' mental health needs, there were still problems. Systemic problems with student discipline and behavior continued to create difficulties with classroom management while also creating barriers to learning and achievement. Likewise, teacher burnout and emotional stress were reported as contributing factors in their ongoing emotional exhaustion (Jennings & Greenberg, 2009). Furthermore, a lack of systematic procedures for evaluating program effectiveness led to inefficiency and redundancy of efforts (Elias et al., 2015).

3.2.1.8 The Need for Social-Emotional Learning in Education

The recognition of effective teaching to students with disabilities is related to but also distinct from addressing social and emotional needs of students. In the nineteenth and twentieth centuries, as education evolved and the world became more industrialized, attention to children's academic and cognitive development became the primary focus of education. The Dewey model of education was designed to serve an industrialized nation, and it continues to exist in the present day, despite it no longer meeting the needs of today's modern society (Hildebrand, 2022). It may be that education's origins in group-level instruction has made it difficult to focus on individual learning needs, especially in the emotional realm. The evidence from neuroscience and other fields has repeatedly confirmed that emotions have enormous implications for how students learn (e.g., see Isen et al., 1987; Jung et al., 2014; Phelps, 2004; Shen et al., 2009). Understanding the connections between cognitive and emotional functions "has the potential to revolutionize our understanding of learning in the context of schools" (Immordino-Yang & Damasio, 2007). Theories of social-emotional learning (SEL) in school settings can be traced to the work of James Comer in 1968 with the New Haven School Intervention Project (Comer, 1980). This was later followed by the work of Elias, Weissberg, and colleagues in 1994 (Elias et al., 1997). Building on this, a plethora of SEL frameworks have emerged, each using different terminology and adding to the already confusing landscape of educational frameworks. With more than 100 SEL frameworks from which schools can choose, it is not surprising that schools are perplexed (Jones, 2017). Despite the overwhelming number of frameworks, however, most schools are familiar with and have adopted the one developed by the Collaborative for Academic, Social, and Emotional Learning (CASEL, n.d.).

3.2.2 *Multitiered System of Supports (MTSS)*

The terms response to intervention (RTI) and multitiered system of supports (MTSS) are sometimes used interchangeably in educational settings and discussion, likely because each state implements federal legislation impacting education using its own vernacular and adjusted processes (Berkeley et al., 2020). In the USA, education is conceived as a local imperative, and primarily under local control, thus creating confusion when educators interact outside of their schools, districts, and states.

ESSA defines the MTSS framework as "a comprehensive continuum of evidence-based, systemic practices to support a rapid response to students' needs, with regular observation to facilitate data-based instructional decision-making" (Office of Elementary and Secondary Education, n.d.). Developed from the earlier response to intervention framework (See Fuchs et al., 2003; Gresham, 2002; Hallahan & Mercer, 2002; National Center on Response to Intervention, 2010), MTSS is a problem-solving, proactive approach for helping to prevent further learning difficulties by intervening quickly with students who may be struggling with academic, social, emotional, or behavioral difficulties. Although MTSS has its origins in the RTI model that was introduced in the No Child Left Behind Act (NCLB) of 2001, it is designed to support a broader approach to intervention by helping organize programs, resources, and supports within an organization so that outcomes can be more effective. It often is conceptualized as a multitiered pyramid with each tier representing a continuum of increasingly intensive interventions and supports. In schools where the MTSS framework has been adopted, there typically are three tiers (Center on Multi-Tiered Systems of Support, n.d.). Tier 1 represents universal interventions, resources, and supports that are provided to all students. The purpose of Tier 1 is to ensure the success of all students and to prevent the need for more intensive interventions. Should any students continue to struggle, however, Tier 2 offers additional, more targeted interventions, resources, and supports. These typically are provided to small groups of students. Should any students continue to struggle at Tier 2, they advance to Tier 3 where additional, more intensive interventions, resources, and supports are provided to individual students. At each tier, students who continue to struggle after being provided with interventions, resources, and supports advance to the next tier.

A major challenge, and perhaps the biggest challenge, that most schools face is at Tier 1 where opportunities for prevention reach the greatest number of students. Unfortunately, most schools typically focus only on identifying struggling students at this tier, rather than on developing a strategic plan for supporting "all" students. In the absence of a strategic plan, there is less of a focus on identifying universal efforts (where it should be) and more of a focus on identifying struggling students. As a result, most of the schools' efforts become focused on Tier 2 interventions (Clayton, 2023). One reason for this is that MTSS is perceived as a referral model mirroring the function of many former RTI models, rather than as a prevention model. This misperception results in a failure to understand that as students advance through the multiple tiers, previous interventions and supports are not discontinued, but they may be changed, and more interventions and/or supports may be added.

The MTSS framework, while it may offer differentiated levels of interventions and supports for students, has limitations in its effectiveness when it comes to addressing barriers to learning (Adelman & Taylor, 2016). Specifically, MTSS as adopted by many schools fails to address the critical need for collaborating and coordinating mental health resources and supports with community partners. These efforts, along with several other foundational components, should be incorporated into every school's processes, but the pragmatics of how MTSS operates in each school will look different. The next section will examine the foundations for developing a successful MTSS framework before moving into a discussion of operating procedures. The section that follows will focus on how schools can organize and align their interventions, supports, and resources using an integrated, whole-child approach.

3.2.2.1 Foundations for Successful MTSS

Establishing the foundations for a successful MTSS framework begins with developing a broad understanding of its underpinnings, which involves several components. These include, but are not limited to, an assets-based philosophy, an equity perspective, use of evidence-based practices, adherence to implementation fidelity, and data-informed decision-making. These substructures play a key role in establishing a successful MTSS foundation, so an explanation of each will preface the discussion of processes and procedures.

An essential underpinning of the MTSS framework is understanding that it operates on an assets-based approach. Instead of identifying student deficits (i.e., a deficits-based approach), an assets-based approach requires that students be viewed as having unique strengths and as able learners who may not have had opportunities to develop and master needed skills. As opposed to the deficits-based approach, an assets-based approach does *not* assume that the problem lies within the student but that the student may have been influenced and motivated by how others have responded to her/him. When the MTSS process employs an assets-based approach, interventions and supports can be organized and aligned with existing school efforts and prevent students from being siloed into specific programs.

As with any educational program, evidence-based practices are recommended (Stoiber & Gettinger, 2016). Unfortunately, adoption of these practices in schools has been slow and uneven, and despite what the research promises, they have not been as successful as when implemented with adequate fidelity and competence (Owens et al., 2014). When schools implement new social, emotional, and behavioral programs, less than half of them are implemented with fidelity, and only one in three is likely to be implemented successfully (Lyon, 2017). A lack of knowledge and understanding of implementation strategies, along with a lack of intentional efforts to employ these strategies, have been recognized as weaknesses (Proctor et al., 2013) and may require that schools provide additional training and coaching of staff to ensure successful implementation.

Compounding the problems with implementation fidelity are concerns over cultural and racial sensitivity when selecting and implementing programs, practices, and interventions. Historically, certain groups of students (especially those from marginalized and minoritized groups) have been excluded from research practices, program development, and piloting of new programs (Venkateswaran et al., 2023). This is especially significant when considering supports and interventions for students who present with behavior and discipline concerns. Disproportionate outcomes for these students are well-documented and has become a critical priority (Davison et al., 2022). Interventions that promote equitable treatment of these students is a vital component of the MTSS process. Therefore, when selecting a new program or intervention, it is recommended that its technical aspects be evaluated prior to implementation. If the new program or intervention includes features that are likely to produce positive outcomes for culturally and linguistically diverse students and can be implemented with fidelity and intention, it may be appropriate for improving the outcomes of all students (Cartledge et al., 2016; Castro-Villarreal et al., 2016; Donovan & Cross, 2002; Harry & Klingner, 2006; Hosp & Madyun, 2007; Losen & Orfield, 2002).

Essential to formulating a successful MTSS process is an effective method for decision-making and ongoing improvement. For the past several decades, the data-driven approach, combined with advances in technology, has influenced schools' decisions about what should be taught and how it should be taught. However, the field of education has struggled to effectively manage and use the data, and this data-driven, decision-making (DDDM) process has come under scrutiny in recent years. Possible explanations for this are a lack of analytic expertise in evaluating the data, difficulty in quantifying some data, and a limited view of data (e.g., failure to view data through a lens of equity and diversity). Consequently, the DDDM process may have contributed to limited or incorrect uses of data in schools. An alternative approach to the use of data in decision-making is to use it to inspire critical thinking. When this approach is used, schools can begin to view data as more than a driver of decisions, but also as a tool that can inform the process or inspire it, especially in evaluating for continuous improvement.

3.2.2.2 Guidelines and Procedures for Implementing MTSS

Following the approach of implementation science, MTSS benefits from several structural and procedural elements:

1. Ensuring diversity and equity in committee membership;
2. Clarifying roles and responsibilities of committee members;
3. Establishing procedures for conducting meetings, prioritizing interventions, collecting data, establishing the fidelity of interventions, and documenting outcomes;
4. Ensuring all interventions and supports are sensitive to diversity and cultural needs; and
5. Identifying the professional development needs related to MTSS and its procedures for all relevant stakeholders.

3.2.2.3 Challenges with Implementing MTSS

The implementation of change in schools is rarely straightforward. Embedding school change in a larger systems change can be even more daunting. Research indicates that implementing change is best supported by a positive school climate, which involves several dimensions. While there is no consensus on which dimensions are most critical, the National Center on Safe Supportive Learning Environments (n.d.) identifies 3 primary domains and 13 subdomains. These are (1) engagement (relationships, cultural and linguistic competence, and school participation), (2) safety (emotional safety, physical safety, bullying/cyberbullying, substance use, and emergency readiness and management), and (3) environment (physical environment, instructional environment, physical health, mental health, and discipline). Understanding how these dimensions are interconnected and interact to create positive and effective learning environments can be challenging but is fundamental to the change process.

Another challenge to implementing the MTSS framework is inconsistent terminology. This framework is not new in public education but has evolved from other multitiered frameworks such as response to intervention (RTI) and schoolwide positive behavioral interventions and supports (SWPBIS). As familiarity with these similar-type frameworks has grown, their acronyms have been used inconsistently and often interchangeably. Because of this, schools struggle with differentiating MTSS and its intended purpose from these other, similar frameworks. Developing a common language around MTSS is frequently the first challenge encountered by schools but is necessary for overcoming confusion, ensuring a common perspective of the issues, and establishing a common vision for implementation.

In addition to the confusion over terminology, MTSS requires a shift in the mindset of how it is viewed by the school's staff. This can be extremely challenging in a system that has traditionally operated from a deficits-based perspective. Instinctively, staff will want to view MTSS as a "clearance route" through which struggling students must pass before being referred to other programs. Thus, schools should plan to devote time and attention to shifting the philosophical thinking of the school community to one that is assets-based instead of deficits-based.

While there may be challenges that are unique to each school, some of the challenges commonly shared by most schools include overcoming budgetary constraints, challenges in assigning roles and responsibilities to the initiative's leaders, and logistical challenges such as problems and conflicts in scheduling meetings, communication issues, allocating staff for data collection, and oversight of the initiative.

3.2.3 Social-Emotional Wellness Under a Tiered Prevention Framework

Given the rising concerns over student mental health, the shortage of mental health service providers in schools, the underfunding of mental health initiatives, and the shrinking availability of community resources for mental health, taking a proactive, preventive approach to addressing these problems may be the most effective and sustaining. One approach that many schools have begun to embrace is social-emotional learning (SEL). Although SEL is not new, some believe it is simply another inconsequential fad in education. Contradicting this belief are volumes of studies and reports suggesting that SEL is more than a fad but is a necessary component of education. In a national survey, teachers not only reported that SEL provides benefits for students' academic, social, emotional, and behavioral development, but they also considered it "the" missing component in education (Bridgeland et al., 2013).

3.3 Integrating Tiered Prevention Frameworks: Social-Emotional Learning (SEL) and MTSS

While many have adopted this framework, there remain confusion and a lack of guidance on how to implement SEL. The following section seeks to provide this guidance through a discussion of how SEL efforts can be integrated with MTSS processes to simultaneously resolve problems with struggling students by using a whole-child approach. Through the coordinated and collaborative processes of MTSS and SEL, the school can address not only the academic needs of students but also their social and emotional needs. Figure 3.2 provides a visual representation of what this process might look like, but it's important to note that every school is unique, so by design, it may look different in every school.

Figure 3.2 illustrates the primary components of an integrated framework. As depicted in the illustration, the SEL framework encompasses the entire school community, which is not confined to the school building but includes the broader community, as well. Within the school community, the SEL framework operates as a guide for infusing social and emotional pedagogy and practices into all aspects of

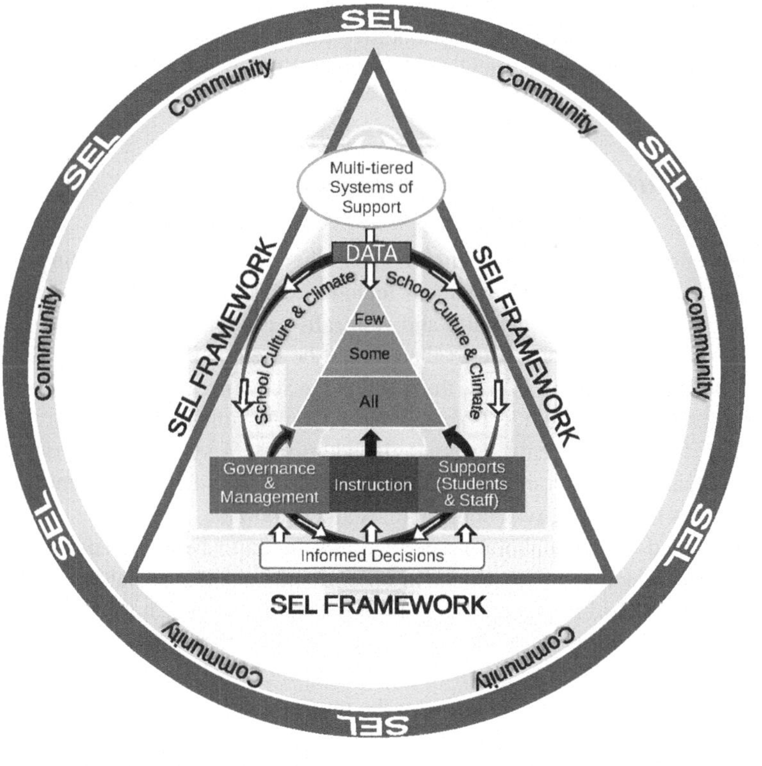

Fig. 3.2 Integrated SEL-MTSS systemwide framework. (Source: Black (2022b). Reprinted with permission of the publisher)

the school's processes, operations, and activities, including the school's culture and climate. The MTSS framework depicted in the center of the illustration is a problem-solving framework that uses data and systematic processes to address and solve problems. This process helps drive all school activities forward, including instruction, governance and management, and identification of all resources and supports. In summary, the MTSS framework serves as the mechanism through which all school efforts move forward, while the SEL framework helps guide those efforts to ensure that social-emotional development remains as important as academic development.

To assist schools with integrating the two frameworks, the Council of Chief State School Officers (CCSSO); the Collaborative for Academic, Social, and Emotional Learning (CASEL); and the American Institutes for Research® (AIR) published the *SEL MTSS Toolkit for State and District Leaders* (2021). The toolkit acknowledges that both frameworks are important for building positive learning conditions that can help young people develop the competencies they need for success in school and throughout life. However, the authors of the toolkit caution schools about trying to advance both frameworks in parallel. Instead, they believe that schools will experience greater success if they intentionally integrate the two frameworks, and in doing so, they are more likely to "build coherence, and to foster a system of support that efficiently – and equitably – addresses the needs of the whole child" (Council of Chief State School Officers, Collaborative for Academic, Social, and Emotional Learning, and American Institutes for Research, 2021, p. 6).

3.3.1 Ensuring Fidelity in Implementation

As noted, adopting new programs in schools is challenging. When selecting a school based SEL program, it's important to include a curriculum of direct, systematic instruction that is developmentally and culturally appropriate. Durlak et al. (2011) identified four training procedures that should be included in a school's SEL program. Using the acronym SAFE, these are (1) a ***S***equenced training approach, (2) ***A***ctive forms of learning, (3) ***F***ocused and adequate time spent on skill development, and (4) ***E***xplicit learning goals. In addition to a systematic curriculum of instruction, an SEL program also should provide opportunities for students to apply learned skills through daily school routines and activities.

Schools and their collaborative partners will need to be knowledgeable of the strategies of implementation science in order to enhance the probability of success and ensure fidelity of implementation. Implementation science has its origins in the medical field and has been defined as "…the scientific study of methods to promote the systematic uptake of research findings and other evidence-based practice into routine practice and, hence, to improve the quality and effectiveness of health services" (Eccles & Mittman, 2006, p. 2). When SEL and MTSS are fully integrated and guided by the strategies of implementation science, not only are the school's chances of improving student outcomes increased but so are their chances of improving system outcomes. When students thrive, so do the systems that serve them.

3.3.2 Two Complementary Frameworks

While the MTSS and SEL frameworks share commonalities and are complementary to one another, they are different in their intended purposes. While both frameworks are prevention models, the primary focus of the MTSS framework is on coordinating and aligning supports, interventions, and resources using a systematic process of decision-making that is informed by data. The primary focus of the SEL framework, however, is on helping students build competencies in social-emotional development, like those promoted by the CASEL framework and often referred to as the "CASEL 5." These include (1) self-awareness, (2) social awareness, (3) self-management, (4) relationship skills, and (5) responsible decision-making (Collaborative for Academic, Social and Emotional Learning, n.d.). Developing students' SEL competencies is equally as important as building their academic competencies. Not only do they help prepare students for success after high school, but they also help build skills that will be needed for success in life, which includes mental health literacy and mental wellness. A successful SEL framework, however, is dependent upon the school's conditions for learning, which includes school culture and climate, pedagogy and practice, governance and management, and supports for students and staff. Creating these supportive conditions in the learning environment can be demanding for schools, but once established, they ensure long-term sustainability of the school's SEL efforts.

To further distinguish these two frameworks, it may be helpful to think of the MTSS framework as the "vehicle" through which the school transports and delivers its services, resources, and supports to its student population. Using data, the school can systematically track and allocate resources, expenses, and outcomes to help make informed decisions. The SEL framework, however, provides the school with a big picture of its "destination." Like a road map for vehicles, the SEL framework helps the school target its goals, chart its journey, and identify the conditions needed to help make the journey safe, efficient, effective, and successful.

Both MTSS and SEL are prevention-focused frameworks that proactively employ a multitiered approach, evidence-based practices, and an assets-based philosophy. When both frameworks are integrated, schools can organize and align their programs and resources to identify the system of supports that are needed at each tier of intervention, with Tiers 1 and 2 focused on preventing more intensive needs. Table 3.1 illustrates this process using a matrix that helps guide schools in organizing and aligning relevant programs, practices, interventions, supports, and resources at each tier to ensure a continuum of supports. After completing the matrix and determining where gaps exist (if any), the school can move forward with implementation.

Table 3.1 SEL-MTSS: matrix for a continuum of integrated supports

MTSS foundations	**Tier 1**	**Tier 2**	**Tier 3**
Student strengths or assets: Identify the frequency and method for instructing, practicing, and evaluating student competencies (at each tier) in all domains of learning (i.e., academic, social, emotional, and behavioral). Identify when, where, and how instruction for social-emotional learning is integrated throughout the school environment and school day. What supports and professional development opportunities are provided to staff in each area?			
Diversity, sensitivity, and culturally responsive practices: Identify programs, interventions, supports, and resources that are provided to students of different ethnicity, race, language, gender, sexual orientation, or religious preference (curricular and extracurricular). Identify which programs and supports are relevant and appropriate to the academic, social, emotional, and behavioral development of these students. Identify any professional development opportunities provided for staff that focus on pedagogy and practice related to diversity, sensitivity, and cultural responsiveness			
Evidence-based practices: Identify evidence-based programs, practices, interventions, resources, and supports that are provided to students (at each tier) in the academic, social, emotional, and behavioral domains of learning. Identify implementation strategies that help ensure fidelity of implementation (e.g., training and coaching, as appropriate, for staff implementing the program/practice; frequency and methods of monitoring implementation; frequency and method of data collection, review, and analysis; etc.). Identify evidence-based programs and practices (at each tier) that have been determined appropriate for marginalized and minoritized students. Identify professional development opportunities for training staff in implementation strategies that are guided by implementation science			
Data-informed decisions: Identify sources of data and how the continuous improvement process is used to inform decisions about the social, emotional, academic, and behavioral needs of *all* students. Which data is used to inspire new and/or innovative practices (e.g., climate surveys, parent needs surveys, student surveys, etc.)? Identify professional development opportunities through which staff have been trained in data review, analysis, interpretation, and use			
SEL conditions for learning	**Tier 1**	**Tier 2**	**Tier 3**
Systemic and explicit instruction of SEL competencies using culturally responsive practices: Identify routines and practices through which SEL competencies are explicitly taught and practiced (e.g., morning meetings, SEL class, etc.). How frequently do these activities occur? Identify routines and practices through which SEL competencies are integrated into the school environment throughout the day and by all staff? Identify any curricular programs and practices that are used for explicit instruction of SEL competencies. Are programs and practices developmentally appropriate, and did they include a diverse student population in their development? Identify pedagogy and practices that are sensitive and responsive to diversity and cultural differences			

(continued)

Table 3.1 (continued)

School connections: Identify how the school has evaluated the culture and climate and how the data is being used to establish safe school environments, build healthy relationships, ensure the physical and emotional safety of *all* students, and encourage school pride and a sense of purpose in *all* students. Identify programs, practices, resources, and supports that encourage engagement of *all* learners (e.g., curricular, extracurricular, service-learning projects, etc.). Identify opportunities through which *all* students have a voice and can provide leadership, as appropriate. Are equitable opportunities afforded to *all* students? Are these opportunities sensitive to diversity and inclusion of *all* students?			
Transitions: Identify supports for in-class transitions, schoolwide transitions, school-to-school transitions, school and home transitions, school and community transitions, and school and college/career transitions for *all* students			
Safety and crises: Identify the school's crisis plan. What are the plans, practices, resources, and supports that focus on preventing crises, planning and preparing for crises, and responding to crises for *all* students? Are the plan, practices, resources, and supports sensitive and responsive to cultural differences, diversity, and equity?			
Family and home engagement: Identify the programs, interventions, resources, and supports that address parent literacy and parent education, as appropriate, in mental health, behavior, academic, and social-emotional development. Identify the school's efforts to involve parents in their child's/children's schooling. Identify how the school provides opportunities, as appropriate, for parents to have a voice in processes, policies, practices, and strategic planning			
School mental health and wellness: Identify programs, practices, and strategies used by the school to ensure the mental health and wellness of *all* students (e.g., bully prevention, safety in the use of technology, peer mentors, coaching, etc.). Which programs, practices, supports, and resources are provided to *all* students, to those who may be at-risk of mental illness, and/or to those who have a mental illness or may have experienced a traumatic life event (e.g., trauma-informed practices, support groups, peer mentors, counseling services, etc.). Identify the school's mental health service providers that are available, as appropriate, to provide intervention support for *all* students and for targeted groups or individual students			
School-community partnerships: Identify the partnerships that the school has developed with community members and/or organizations that provide (1) mentoring, (2) volunteering, (3) opportunities for recreational enrichment or remedial supports, (4) nutritional supports, (5) social services, and (6) access to mental health and/or public health services. Identify which of these resources and supports are available to *all* students, targeted groups of students, and individual students			

This matrix is designed to help schools organize all programs, practices, interventions, resources, supports, and staff professional development opportunities. Once these have been organized, any gaps in specific areas or tiers can be identified. One suggested approach for completing the matrix is to create a pyramid on a large drawing board and address each specific area within the tier that it falls

3.3.3 Implementation as a Process, Not a Program

When implementing the SEL-MTSS framework, it is helpful if school personnel understand that implementation is a process, not a program, and it requires a multiyear, multiphase approach and a strategic plan. Implementation should not be the responsibility of any single person or position but requires everyone's commitment and support. Determining a school's readiness for implementation is a critical initial first step and likely will affect the long-term sustainability of the program (Meyers et al., 2012; Wanless & Domitrovich, 2015). While teachers may support SEL and the benefits it offers (Collie et al., 2012), school leaders should not assume they will understand the complexities of implementation and be ready to teach SEL competencies. SEL necessitates that teachers (even those who are supportive of the initiative) be given special preparation before being required to implement an SEL curriculum (Schonert-Reichl et al., 2017).

The SEL-MTSS framework is *not* intended to be a "one-size-fits-all" framework but must be tailored to meet the unique needs of each school in which it is implemented. Every school community is different, so the framework will look different in each school. The success of implementation will be contingent upon how well the school identifies its unique needs. Identifying needs starts with a self-review, followed by a reflection on what needs to be improved.

3.3.4 Implementation Requires Strategic Planning

A strategic plan for implementing the SEL-MTSS framework should include a system of program evaluation that is driven by a theory of change. This process begins with an examination of the school's accountability data but also includes a comprehensive review of systems, programs, learning needs, and supports. Schools are strongly advised to have baseline information to guide their improvement efforts. Figure 3.3 provides a visual illustration of a tool designed specifically for this purpose and reprinted with permission of the publisher.

Once the information from each group has been collected and reviewed, a self-portrait of the school emerges that can be used to identify targeted areas where improvement is needed. While a large focus of a school's plan will likely be on student support systems, schools should not neglect the need for teacher support systems, especially in the area of professional development. The demands of teaching in today's complex education system necessitates that teachers be given professional development opportunities that allow them to provide a quality education to students. Only half (50.9%) of the teacher workforce in the USA report they have been released from teaching to attend professional development opportunities. Of these, fewer than a third (28.2%) were reimbursed for conference or workshop fees (Garcia & Weiss, 2019). Considering these findings, schools will need to ensure opportunities for professional development when developing their implementation

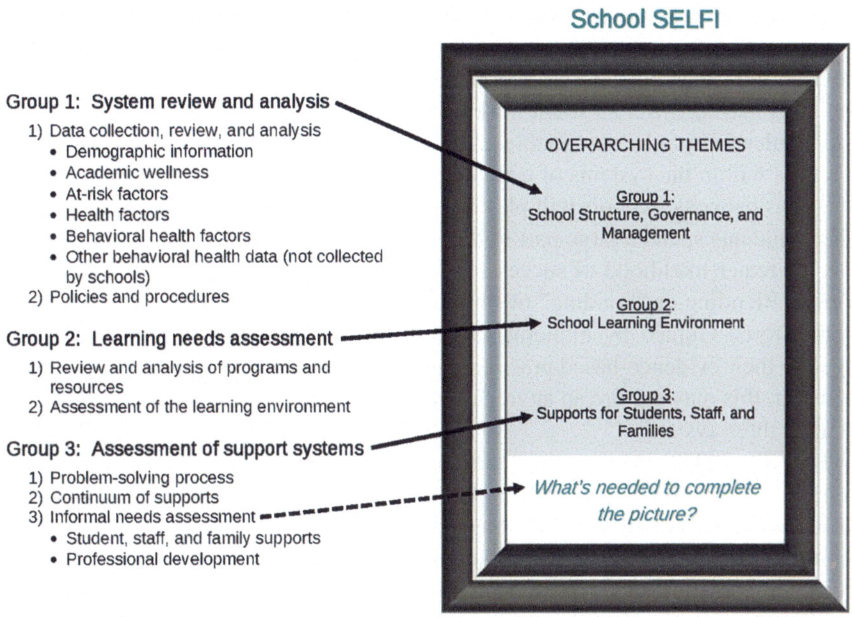

Fig. 3.3 The Social-Emotional Learning Foundations Inventory (SELFI). (Source: Black (2022c). Reprinted with permission of the publisher)

and strategic improvement plans. Critical areas should include mental health literacy and SEL instructional competency, among others. Research suggests that improving teachers' mental health literacy can help improve mental health promotion and prevention in schools (Kutcher & Wei, 2013; Simkiss et al., 2020). Likewise, professional development opportunities that help teachers develop SEL instructional competency, especially from an equity, diversity, and culturally responsive perspective, can improve teacher job satisfaction and increase teacher retention in schools (Soutter, 2023).

3.4 Conclusion

In 2021, US Surgeon General Vivek Murthy issued an advisory report regarding the dire state of children's mental health in America. In the report, it was noted that the prevalence of mental health challenges in young people already was at crises levels before the COVID-19 pandemic but since then had only worsened (U.S. Surgeon General, 2021). Schools have attempted to address these challenges, but inconsistent funding and shortages of mental health professionals have limited their efforts (National Center for Education Statistics, 2022). These barriers, rising mental health problems, underfunding of mental health resources, and critical shortages in mental health service providers, have come together to form a public health crisis.

The education sector and local schools have been particularly vulnerable to the negative effects of rampant mental health challenges. There is reason to believe that the need for robust prevention-focused solutions is greater now than has ever been. An integrated SEL-MTSS framework offers a promising solution for this problem, but in order for it to be sustainable, there must be a convergence in thinking and in practices within the systems of education, mental health, and public health. If and when this happens, schools will play a vital role in the process because schools are where students spend a large part of their time and schools are where interventions have a greater likelihood of success. Of course, funding to support such efforts is critical. Blending or "braiding" of funds and services may be necessary to support these efforts. Guided by implementation science, these three systems must join together their evidence-based practices and help close the research-to-practice gap. However, this may require an aggregation of knowledge, experience, and resources from all three systems.

The SEL-MTSS integrated framework offers a viable, sustainable mechanism through which schools can address the social, emotional, academic, and behavioral health needs of all students, thus reducing the need for more intensive mental health supports. Although this approach is an evidence-based practice and reduces the need for high level services when implemented correctly, schools cannot, and should not, bear responsibility for the mental health crisis alone. Developing and advancing an initiative of this magnitude requires a strategic plan that needs to include stakeholders and collaborative partners within the broader systems level (district, region, and/or state). This would include parents, community members, policymakers, members of the faith-based community, representatives of other child-serving agencies, and members of the mental health and public health fields, among others. Through an alliance with these partners and a sharing of resources and efforts, the likelihood of success and sustainability is significantly strengthened.

Competing Interests *The author has no conflicts of interest to declare that are relevant to the content of this chapter.*

References

Adelman, H., & Taylor, L. (2005). *The implementation guide to student learning supports in the classroom and schoolwide*. Corwin Press.

Adelman, H., & Taylor, L. (2016, October). *ESSA state consolidated plans: Rethinking MTSS to better address barriers to learning*. Research for School Improvement and Transformation from the National Center for Mental Health in Schools in the Department of Psychology at UCLA. https://smhp.psych.ucla.edu/pdfdocs/essamtss.pdf

American Academy of Pediatrics, American Academy of Child and Adolescent Psychiatry, and Children's Hospital Association. (2021, October). *AAP-AACAP-CHA declaration of a national emergency in child and adolescent mental health*. https://www.aap.org/en/advocacy/child-and-adolescent-healthy-mental-development/aap-aacap-cha-declaration-of-a-national-emergency-in-child-and-adolescent-mental-health/

American School Counselor Association. (2019). *The ASCA national model: A framework for school counseling programs* (4th ed.). ASCA.

American School Counselor Association. (2023, September). *Current issues in education: School counselor shortages*. https://www.schoolcounselor.org/getmedia/f73304ab-5ac5-4ba5-8342-826a3bc205a2/CIE-Employment-Shortages.pdf

Araújo, L., Veloso, C., Souza, M., Azevedo, J., & Tarro, G. (2021). The potential impact of the COVID-19 pandemic on child growth and development: A systematic review. *Jornal de Pediatria, 97*(4), 369–377. https://doi.org/10.1016/j.jped.2020.08.008

Aspen Institute. (n.d.). *Aspen Institute's education and society program: A rich vision for public education*. Retrieved February 10, 2024, from https://www.aspeninstitute.org/programs/education-and-society-program/principal-2/

Berkeley, S., Scanlon, D., Bailey, T. R., Sutton, J. C., & Sacco, D. M. (2020). A snapshot of RTI implementation a decade later: New picture, same story. *Journal of Learning Disabilities, 53*(5), 332–342.

Black, D. (2022b). Getting started: A multiphase approach to whole school implementation of SEL. In A. Kaufman & N. Kaufman (Eds.), *Essentials of social emotional learning (SEL): The complete guide for schools and practitioners*. Wiley.

Black, D. (2022a). Making the case for SEL. In A. Kaufman & N. Kaufman (Eds.), *Essentials of social emotional learning (SEL): The complete guide for schools and practitioners*. Wiley.

Black, D. (2022c). Tools, templates, and checklists. In A. Kaufman & N. Kaufman (Eds.), *Essentials of social emotional learning (SEL): The complete guide for schools and practitioners*. Wiley.

Bridgeland, J., Bruce, M., & Hariharan, A. (2013). *The missing piece: A national teacher survey on how social and emotional learning can empower children and transform schools*. Civic Enterprises, Peter D. Hart Research Associates, & Collaborative for Academic, Social, and Emotional Learning. https://www.edu-links.org/sites/default/files/media/file/the-missing-piece.pdf

Burr, R., Kemp, J., & Wang, K. (2024). *Crime, violence, discipline, and safety in U.S. public schools: Findings from the school survey on crime and safety: 2021–22 (NCES 2024-043)*. U.S. Department of Education, National Center for Education Statistics. Retrieved March 20, 2024, from https://nces.ed.gov/pubsearch/pubsinfo.asp?pubid=2024043

Cartledge, G., Kea, C. D., Watson, M., & Oif, A. (2016). Special education disproportionality: A review of response to intervention and culturally relevant pedagogy. *Multiple Voices for Ethnically Diverse Exceptional Learners, 16*(1), 29–49.

Castro-Villarreal, F., Villarreal, V., & Sullivan, J. R. (2016). Special education policy and response to intervention: Identifying promises and pitfalls to advance social justice for diverse students. *Contemporary School Psychology, 20*, 10–20. https://doi.org/10.1007/s40688015-0077-3

Center on Multi-Tiered Systems of Support. (n.d.). *Essential components of MTSS*. https://mtss4success.org/essential-components

Clayton, J. (2023, December). Navigating the practical challenges of MTSS implementation. *Communiqué, 52*(4), 12–16.

Collaborative for Academic, Social, an Emotional Learning (CASEL). (n.d.). *What is the CASEL framework?* https://casel.org/fundamentals-of-sel/what-is-the-casel-framework/

Collie, R., Shapka, J., & Perry, N. (2012). School climate and social–emotional learning: Predicting teacher stress, job satisfaction, and teaching efficacy. *Journal of Educational Psychology, 104*(4), 1189–1204. https://doi.org/10.1037/a0029356

Comer, J. (1980, June 5). *The New Haven school intervention project* [Paper presentation]. Strategies for Urban School Improvement Workshop Series, Washington, DC, USA.

Council of Chief State School Officers, Collaborative for Academic, Social, and Emotional Learning, and American Institutes for Research. (2021). *SEL MTSS toolkit for state and district leaders*. Council of Chief State School Officers. https://753a0706.flowpaper.com/CCSSOSELMTSSToolkit/#page=1

Davison, M., Penner, A., & Penner, E. (2022). Restorative for all? Racial disproportionality and school discipline under restorative justice. *American Educational Research Journal, 59*(4), 687–718. https://doi.org/10.3102/00028312211062613

Donovan, S. M., & Cross, C. T. (2002). *Minority students in special and gifted education*. National Academies Press.

Durlak, J. A., Weissberg, R. P., Dymnicki, A. B., Taylor, R. D., & Schellinger, K. B. (2011). The impact of enhancing students' social and emotional learning: A meta-analysis of school-based universal interventions. *Child Development, 82*, 405–432. https://doi.org/10.1111/j.1467-8624.2010.01564.x

Eccles, M., & Mittman, B. (2006). Welcome to implementation science. *Implementation Science, 1*(1). https://doi.org/10.1186/1748-5908-1-1

Elias, M. J., Zins, J. E., Weissberg, R. P., Frey, K. S., Greenberg, M. T., Haynes, N. M., Kessler, R., Schwab-Stone, M. E., & Shriver, T. P. (1997). Promoting social and emotional learning: Guidelines for educators. *Association for Supervision and Curriculum Development.*

Elias, M. J., Leverett, L., Duffell, J., Humphrey, N., Stepney, C. T., & Ferrito, J. J. (2015). Integrating social-emotional learning with related prevention and youth-development approaches. In J. A. Durlak, C. Domitrovich, R. P. Weissberg, T. P. Gullotta, & T. (Eds.), *Handbook of social and emotional learning (SEL): Research and practice* (pp. 33–49). The Guilford Press.

Exec. Order No. 13227, 3 C.F.R. 51287-51289. (2001). https://www.federalregister.gov/documents/2001/10/05/01-25344/presidents-commission-on-excellence-in-special-education

Finn, C., Rotherham, A., & Hokanson, C. (Eds.). (2001). *Rethinking special education for a new century*. Fordham Foundation.

Francois, E. J. (2015). *Building global education with a local perspective*. Palgrave Macmillan. https://doi.org/10.1057/9781137386779_1

Fuchs, D., Mock, D., Morgan, P. L., & Young, C. L. (2003). Responsiveness-to-intervention: Definitions, evidence, and implications for the learning disabilities construct. *Learning Disabilities Research & Practice, 18*, 157–171.

Garcia, E. & Weiss, E. (2019, July 26). Teachers need better professional development opportunities, more support. Economic Policy Institute. https://www.epi.org/blog/teachers-need-better-professional-development-opportunities-more-support-from-the-system/

Goldhaber, D., Kane, T., McEachin, A., Morton, E., Patterson, T., & Staiger, D. (2022). *The consequences of remote and hybrid instruction during the pandemic*. Center for Education Policy Research, Harvard University. https://cepr.harvard.edu/files/cepr/files/5-4.pdf?m=1651690491

Gresham, F. M. (2002). Responsiveness to intervention: An alternative approach to the identification of learning disabilities. In R. Bradley, L. Danielson, & D. P. Hallahan (Eds.), *Identification of learning disabilities*. Lawrence Erlbaum Associates.

Hallahan, D. P., & Mercer, C. D. (2002). Learning disabilities: Historical perspectives. In R. Bradley, L. Danielson, & D. P. Hallahan (Eds.), *Identification of learning disabilities* (pp. 1–67). Lawrence Erlbaum Associates.

Harry, B., & Klingner, J. (2006). *Why are so many minority students in special education? Understanding race and disability in schools*. Teachers College Press.

Health Resources and Services Administration. (2024, March 31). *Designated health professional shortage areas statistics*. https://data.hrsa.gov/topics/health-workforce/shortage-areas

Hildebrand, D. L. (2022). John Dewey. In *The Routledge companion to pragmatism* (pp. 26–34). Routledge.

Hosp, J. L., & Madyun, N. H. (2007). Addressing disproportionality with response to intervention. In S. R. Jimerson, M. K. Burns, & A. M. VanDerHeyden (Eds.), *Handbook of response to intervention* (pp. 172–181). Springer. https://doi.org/10.1007/978-0-387-49053-3

Immordino-Yang, M., & Damasio, A. (2007). We feel therefore we learn: The relevance of affective and social neuroscience to education. *Mind, Brain, and Education, 1*(1), 3–10.

Individuals with Disabilities Education Act. (2024, February 6). *Wikipedia*. https://en.wikipedia.org/wiki/Individuals_with_Disabilities_Education_Act

Individuals with Disabilities Education Act. (n.d.). *A history of the Individuals with Disabilities Education Act*. Retrieved February 20, 2024, from https://sites.ed.gov/idea/IDEA-History

Isen, A. M., Daubman, K. A., & Nowicki, G. P. (1987). Positive affect facilitates creative problem solving. *Journal of Personality and Social Psychology, 52*, 1122–1131. https://doi.org/10.1037/0022-3514.52.6.1122

Jennings, P., & Greenberg, M. (2009). The prosocial classroom: Teacher social and emotional competence in relation to student and classroom outcomes. *Review of Educational Research, 79*(1), 491–525. https://journals.sagepub.com/doi/10.3102.003465430832593

Jones, S. (2017). Harvard graduate school of education. *The Taxonomy Project*. https://easel.gse.harvard.edu/taxonomy-project

Jung, N., Wranke, C., Hamburger, K., & Knauff, M. (2014). How emotions affect logical reasoning: Evidence from experiments with mood-manipulated participants, spider phobics, and people with exam anxiety. *Frontiers in Psychology, 5*, 570. https://doi.org/10.3389/fpsyg.2014.00570

Kutcher, S., & Wei, Y. (2013). Educator mental health literacy: A programme evaluation of the teacher training education on the mental health & high school curriculum guide. *Advances in School Mental Health Promotion, 6*(2), 83–93. https://doi.org/10.1080/1754730X.2013.784615

Landrum, T., & Kauffman, J. (n.d.). *Education of emotionally disturbed*. https://education.stateuniversity.com/pages/1952/Emotionally-Disturbed-Education.html

Losen, D. J., & Orfield, G. (2002). *Racial inequity in special education*. Harvard Education Publishing Group.

Lyon, A. (2017). *Implementation science and practice in the education sector* (Issue Brief No. 072617). Substance Abuse and Mental Health Services Administration and Project Aware. http://files.constantcontact.com/bde05f96001/bf06f755-5ae6-4c31-8373-d7b41affe7dc.pdf

Mahomed, F. (2020). Addressing the problem of severe underinvestment in mental health and well-being from a human rights perspective. *Health and Human Rights, 22*(1), 35–49. https://www.ncbi.nlm.nih.gov/pmc/articles/PMC7348439/pdf/hhr-22-01-035.pdf

Meyers, D. C., Durlak, J. A., & Wandersman, A. (2012). The quality implementation framework: A synthesis of critical steps in the implementation process. *American Journal of Community Psychology, 50*(3–4), 462–480. https://doi.org/10.1007/s10464-012-9522-x

National Academies of Sciences, Engineering, and Medicine. (2023). *Addressing the long-term effects of the COVID-19 pandemic on children and families*. The National Academies Press. https://doi.org/10.17226/26809

National Association of School Psychologists. (n.d.). *Shortage of school psychologists*. https://www.nasponline.org/research-and-policy/policy-priorities/critical-policy-issues/shortage-of-school-psychologists

National Center for Education Statistics. (2022). *Prevalence of mental health services provided by public schools and limitations in schools' efforts to provide mental health services. Condition of Education*. U.S. Department of Education, Institute of Education Sciences. Retrieved April 24, 2024, from https://nces.ed.gov/programs/coe/indicator/a23

National Center on Response to Intervention (NCRTI). (2010, March). *Essential components of RTI—A closer look at response to intervention*. U.S. Department of Education, Office of Special Education Programs, National Center on Response to Intervention.

National Center on Safe Supportive Learning Environments. (n.d.). *School climate improvement*. https://safesupportivelearning.ed.gov/school climate-improvement

Newman, L., Wagner, M., Cameto, R., & Knokey, A.-M. (2009). *The post-high school outcomes of youth with disabilities up to four years after high school. A report from the National Longitudinal Transition Study-2 (NLTS2) (NCSER 2009-3017)*. http://ies.ed.gov/ncser/pdf/20093017.pdf

No Child Left Behind Act (NCLB) of 2001. 20 U.S.C. § 6301 *et.seq.* (2001). https://www.congress.gov/bill/107th-congress/house-bill/1/text

Office of Disability Employment Policy. (2023, July 26). *Examining 50 years of the Rehabilitation Act of 1973—Section 504*. U.S. Department of Labor Blog. https://blog.dol.gov/2023/07/26/examining-50-years-of-the-rehabilitation-act-of-1973-section-504

Office of Disability Employment Policy. (n.d.). *Braiding, blending, and sequencing*. Retrieved February 20, 2024, from https://www.dol.gov/agencies/odep/program-areas/bbs
Office of Elementary & Secondary Education. (n.d.). *ESSA legislation table of contents*. Retrieved February 11, 2024, from https://oese.ed.gov/offices/office-of-formula-grants/school-support-and-accountability/essa-legislation-table-contents/
Owens, J., Lyon, A., Brandt, N., Warner, C., Nadeem, E., Spiel, C., & Wagner, M. (2014). Implementation science in school mental health: Key constructs in a developing research agenda. *School Mental Health, 6*(2), 99–111. https://doi.org/10.1007/s12310-013-9115-3
Phelps, E. A. (2004). Human emotion and memory: Interactions of the amygdala and hippocampal complex. *Current Opinion in Neurobiology, 14*, 198–202. https://doi.org/10.1016/j.conb.2004.03.015
President's Commission on Excellence in Special Education. (2002). *A new era: Revitalizing special education for children and their families*. https://eric.ed.gov/?id=ED473830
Proctor, E., Powell, B., & McMillen, J. (2013). Implementation strategies: Recommendations for specifying and reporting. *Implementation Science, 8*, 1–11.
Schonert-Reichl, K. A., Kitil, M. J., & Hanson-Peterson, J. (2017). *To reach the students, teach the teachers: A national scan of teacher preparation and social and emotional learning*. A report prepared for the Collaborative for Academic, Social, and Emotional Learning [CASEL]. University of British Columbia. https://casel.org/to-reach-the-students-teach-the-teachers/?view=true
Scott, J., Yellowlees, P., Becker, D. F., & Chen, C. (2023). Virtual care and mental health: Dismantling silos to strengthen care delivery. *Telemedicine Reports, 4*(1), 174–179. https://doi.org/10.1089/tmr.2023.0016
Shen, L., Wang, M., & Shen, R. (2009). Affective e-learning: Using "emotional" data to improve learning in pervasive learning environment. *Educational Technology & Society, 12*, 176–189.
Simkiss, N. J., Gray, N. S., Malone, G., Kemp, A., & Snowden, R. J. (2020). Improving mental health literacy in year 9 high school children across Wales: A protocol for a randomised control treatment trial (RCT) of a mental health literacy programme across an entire country. *BMC Public Health, 20*(1), 727. https://doi.org/10.1186/s12889-020-08736-z
Soutter, M. (2023). Transformative social–emotional learning for teachers: Critical and holistic well-being as a marker of success. *Journal of Teaching and Learning, 17*(1), 7–30. https://doi.org/10.22329/jtl.v17i1.7001
Special Education in the United States. (2024, February 6). *Wikipedia*. https://en.wikipedia.org/wiki/Special_education_in_the_United_States#cite_ref-Esteves_and_Rao_1_1-0
Stoiber, K., & Gettinger, M. (2016). Multi-tiered systems of support and evidence-based practices. In S. Jimerson, M. Burns, & A. VanDerHeyden (Eds.), *Handbook of response to intervention* (2nd ed., pp. 121–141). Springer. https://doi.org/10.1007/978-1-4899-7568-3_9
U.S. Department of Education. (2017). *Transitioning to the Every Student Succeeds Act: Frequently asked questions*. https://www.congress.gov/114/plaws/publ95/PLAW-114publ95.pdf
U.S. Department of Education. (2023, February 16). *U.S. Department of Education Announces More Than $188 Million from the Bipartisan Safer Communities Act to Support Mental Health and Student Wellness* [Press release]. https://www.ed.gov/news/press-releases/us-department-education-announces-more-188-million-bipartisan-safer-communities-act-support-mental-health-and-student-wellness
U.S. Department of Education. (n.d.-a). *About IDEA*. Retrieved February 6, 2024, from https://sites.ed.gov/idea/about-idea/#IDEA
U.S. Department of Education. (n.d.-b). *Every Student Succeeds Act (ESSA): A new education law*. Retrieved February 10, 2024, from https://www.ed.gov/essa?src%3Drn
U.S. Surgeon General. (2021). *Protecting youth mental health: The U.S. Surgeon General's advisory*. https://www.hhs.gov/sites/default/files/surgeon-general-youth-mental-health-advisory.pdf?null
United Nations. (2020). *The impact of COVID-19 on children* [Policy brief]. United Nations Secretary General. https://violenceagainstchildren.un.org/content/united-nations-secretary-general-policy-brief-impact-covid-19-children

Venkateswaran, N., Feldman, J., Hawkins, S., Lewis, M., Armstrong-Brown, J., Comfort, M., Lowe, A., & Pineda, D. (2023). *Bringing an equity-centered framework to research: Transforming the researcher, research content, and practice of research* (RTI Press Publication No. OP-0085-2301). RTI Press. https://doi.org/10.3768/rtipress.2023.op.0085.2301

Wanless, S., & Domitrovich, C. (2015). Readiness to implement school-based social-emotional learning interventions: Using research on factors related to implementation to maximize quality. *Prevention Science, 16*, 1037–1043. https://doi.org/10.1007/s11121-015-0612-5

Warren, R. P. (1961). *The legacy of the Civil War* (p. 100). University of Nebraska Press.

Weist, M., Hoover, S., Daly, B., Short, K., & Bruns, E. (2023). Propelling the global advancement of school mental health. *Clinical Child and Family Psychology Review, 26*(4), 851–864. https://doi.org/10.1007/s10567-023-00434-7

World Health Organization (WHO). (2023). *How school systems can improve health and well-being*. https://www.who.int/publications/i/item/9789240064751

Chapter 4
Systems Change: Constructing an Adolescent Public Mental Health Model

Patricia Gail Bray and Arthur Maerlender

4.1 Introduction

This chapter addresses the rationale or *why* systems change for adolescent mental health (AMH) is needed. The intent of this chapter is not to elaborate or reformulate the adolescent mental health problem or to design new programmatic interventions. Rather, the purpose is to shift the lens away from defining the problem and instead focus on providing a framework for possible solutions, whose components are already working somewhat interdependently and are in existence around the world. In this chapter, we provide a brief overview about why current approaches to AMH remain a challenge. Despite global and US declarations and calls to action, the AMH crisis continues to be intractable. Based on the interconnections of three core systems, including the AMH system, along with the public health and school health systems, a call for systems change along with five principles, integrated into a new *adolescent public mental health* (APMH) model, is proposed.

Complex and multiple interpersonal and societal elements that separately and collectively support an unsatisfactory AMH status quo will be addressed. According to Fazel and Soneson (2023), these include the parental, family, community, and societal elements that influence, support, and impact adolescent growth during a critical developmental time. Additionally, creating new and innovative systems

P. G. Bray (✉)
Department of Management, Policy and Community Health, UTHealth Houston School of Public Health, The University of Texas Health Science Center (UTHealth) at Houston, Houston, TX, USA
e-mail: Patricia.G.Bray@uth.tmc.edu

A. Maerlender
Department of Psychology, Saint Anselm College, Manchester, NH, USA

Center for Brain, Biology and Behavior, University of Nebraska—Lincoln, Lincoln, NE, USA
e-mail: amaerlender@anselm.edu

P. G. Bray, A. Maerlender (eds.), *Adolescent Public Mental Health*,
https://doi.org/10.1007/978-3-031-68294-0_4

should necessarily address contextual factors within these elements, such as culture, existing institutions (schools) and organizations, and the AMH social, economic, and political factors. These nonmedical factors are called the social determinants of health and play a significant role in the growth and development of adolescents and have been underutilized in the AMH system.

What is clear is that most of the societal problems experienced by adolescents before, during, and after the pandemic are not limited to an independent, standalone AMH system. Other systems overlap on a daily basis with the health and well-being of adolescents (Murthy, 2021). From a macro perspective, the two systems which are most relevant and interconnected to adolescent mental health are public health and education. Integrating the interconnections among these three systems can result in a systems change for AMH.

The proposed model *adolescent public mental health* (APMH) is based on a multiyear pilot project in Houston, Texas (See Chap. 6 for the full case study discussion). An evidence-based intervention model, the components include adapting a "public health approach" to adolescent mental health (Hurst et al., 2024.) A public health approach includes the integration of the social determinants of health (Marmot & Wilkinson, 1999) and the three prevention tiers of the Institute of Medicine's (1994) mental health continuum model, which includes primary, secondary, and tertiary prevention. Coupled with a multisector approach to collaboration, the APMH model serves to integrate the applicable interconnections between the three AMH, public health, and education systems. As a result of the global COVID-19 pandemic, all systems were affected and increased the challenges for the world's 1.3 billion adolescents (UNICEF, 2023).

The guidelines drawn from implementation science provide direction for addressing the barriers facing evidence-based interventions and practices inherent across these multiple systems (Bauer & Kirchner, 2020). Since implementation science can span the three different systems, strategies can be adapted to help increase the "uptake" of evidence-based innovations.

4.2 Why Does Adolescent Mental Health Remain a Challenge?

4.2.1 Adolescent Prevalence Overview

Scientific research spanning over a century has underscored the profound and enduring impact of pivotal milestones experienced during adolescence (Hall, 1904; Healy, 1915). The term "adolescence" was included in the American Academy of Pediatrics from the founding in 1930, as noted: "[t]he practice of pediatrics begins at birth and should extend through the adolescent period" (American Academy of Pediatrics, 2024). Yet, in the USA, the expanded designation of the American Academy of Child and *Adolescent* Psychiatry did not occur until decades later in

1988 (emphasis added) (American Academy of Child & Adolescent Psychiatry, n.d.). This was followed a few years later, in 1991, when adolescence became formalized as a board-certified subspecialty in medicine in the USA (Lee et al., 2016).

Similarly, progress in translating adolescent mental health knowledge into action has historically been sluggish and compartmentalized, with limited attention until the end of the twentieth century. In 1977 the World Health Organization (WHO) published a seminal report about adolescents, which included the factors affecting physical and psychological health (World Health Organization, 1977, p. 21). Yet, research on the global burden of adolescent mental health disorders received little attention until 2010, when the Global Burden of Disease study investigated mental and substance disorders for youth aged 0–24 years (Erskine et al., 2015).

Adolescent mental health prevalence research increased dramatically in the USA and globally during and after COVID-19. A watershed moment occurred in 2021, when much attention was focused on the adolescent mental health crisis. UNICEF (2021) noted that depression and anxiety constituted 40% of diagnosed mental health disorders globally. A sampling of some of the studies revealed that rates of adolescent depression, anxiety, and suicide had increased. For example, a meta-analysis reviewing 29 studies covering 80,879 youth found that global prevalence for depression and anxiety in children doubled during the COVID-19 pandemic (Racine et al., 2021). The depression and anxiety rates soared to 25.2% and 20.5%, respectively. Another review examining the COVID-19 impact globally on adolescent mental health found increased depression, anxiety, and other forms of psychological distress, comprising burdensomeness, belongingness, stress, trauma, and drug abuse (Jones et al., 2021).

According to the Agency for Healthcare Research and Quality (2022), girls aged 12–17 have experienced a sharp and sustained increase in depression cases since 2009. Another study corroborated the disturbing trend with girls. In a review of emergency department data in Spain after the start of the pandemic, researchers found that adolescent suicide ideation increased significantly, especially for girls during the second year of the pandemic in 2021 (García-Fernández et al., 2023).

In one study published on adolescent suicide behaviors from 90 countries, one of the key findings found that suicide ideation was dramatically higher for girls than for boys, aged 13–17 (Campisi et al., 2020). The WHO (2021) identified suicide as the fourth leading cause of death globally among adolescents aged 15–19. UNICEF (2021) reported that suicide is the fifth most prevalent cause of death for adolescent boys and girls aged 10–19. An estimated 45,800 adolescents die from suicide each year, or more than one person every 11 minutes (UNICEF, 2021). In the USA, suicide for 12–17-year-old adolescents increased by 70.3% between 2008 and 2020, rising from 3.7 to 6.3 deaths per 100,000 (AHRQ, 2022). The highest rate is for White adolescents at 7.4 per 100,000 per population, compared to Hispanics at 5.0 and Black adolescents, 4.6 (AHRQ, 2022). In 2021, the Centers for Disease Control and Prevention (CDC) announced that in the USA, suicide ranks as the second leading cause of death among individuals between the ages of 10–14 and 25–34 and the third leading cause of death for youth ages 15–24 (CDC, 2021; Curtin & Garnett, 2023; Ehlman et al., 2022).

In 2021, 54% (26,328) of all gun-related deaths in the USA were suicides (Gramlich, 2023b). In the USA, between 2019 and 2021, 2590 children and teens under 18 died from gun deaths, representing a 50% increase in those 2 years (Gramlich, 2023a). The USA has the highest rate of gun deaths among peer countries for children and teens ages 1–19 years (KFF, 2023).

4.3 Crisis Declarations and Calls to Action

The alarming evidence revealed prior to and during COVID-19 advanced an AMH urgency. Consequently, a number of key US government and professional organizations officially declared an adolescent mental health crisis (Murthy, 2021; American Academy of Pediatrics, American Academy of Child and Adolescent Psychiatry, & The Children's Hospital Association, 2021). The Agency for Healthcare Quality and Research (2022) noted that data from the announcements of the other professional associations supported the findings of the Surgeon General's advisory regarding the adolescent mental health crisis. Additionally, 130 national and state organizations collectively supported the declaration of a national state of emergency in children's mental health and urged the President to declare a federal national emergency in children's mental health (AAP, 2022).

Globally, reports from the WHO, UNICEF, and others over the past 10 years have featured evidence for the need to take action with the aim to improve the ongoing AMH challenge. Examples of these reports are included in Box 4.1.

Box 4.1: Global Calls to Action for Adolescent Mental Health

- *Health for the World's Adolescents: A Second Chance in the Second Decade* report (World Health Organization, 2014). This report presents a high-level overview of the evidence needed to take action for the crucial adolescent years. A range of issues is discussed, including adolescent mental health.
- *Our Future: A Lancet Commission on Adolescent Health and Wellbeing.* (The Lancet, 2016). This report claims that adolescents and young adults have been overlooked in global health and social policy. One of the goals of the report is to bring global convergence in health to all countries by 2030.
- *Global Accelerated Action for the Health of Adolescents* (AA-HA!): *Guidance to Support Country Implementation* (World Health Organization, 2017). This report outlines the guidance needed to translate the global strategy into action for adolescent health. The recognition of disproportionate risks, including poor physical and mental health, harassment, assault, and rape for adolescents, is considered.

(continued)

Box 4.1 (continued)

- *Adolescent Mental Health: Time for Action* (2019). This is the first joint report from the WHO and UNICEF, and others focused solely on child mental health. Included are multisectoral strategies and interventions for adolescent mental health, ranging from individual psychosocial support, families providing responsive caregiving and emotional connections with families, promotion of adolescent mental health awareness and literacy within schools and communities, and policies to promote optimal adolescent mental health through systems and structures.
- A recent report, *Guidelines on Mental Health Promotive and Preventive Interventions for Adolescents: Helping Adolescents Thrive (HAT)* (World Health Organization, 2020). The themes and principles presented in this volume align with the "evidence-informed recommendations for psychosocial interventions to promote mental health, prevent mental disorders, and reduce self-harm and other risk behaviors among adolescents." These include the complex social, cultural, and economic environments that affect mental health.
- *The State of the World's Children on My Mind: Promoting, Protecting, and Caring for Children's Mental Health* (UNICEF, 2021). Included is a multisector intervention approach with families, schools, and communities to help promote and protect mental health. There are 14 Calls to Action for strengthening children across these sectors within an action framework to commit, communicate and act.

4.4 A New Call to Action for an Adolescent Mental Health Systems Change

4.4.1 Adolescent Mental Health Structural and Systems Challenges

Mental health issues before and during COVID-19 were the leading cause of disability and poor life outcomes (AHRQ, 2022, p. 74; WHO, 2021). With this accumulating evidence about the seriousness of the problem, research on adolescent mental health increased, along with a plethora of innovative programs offering possible solutions. Yet, the seemingly problematic AMH crisis continues to elude scalable and sustainable corrections. The question of why the adolescent mental health challenges have escalated is not a simple one to answer. A recent shift in the literature makes the argument that public health is moving away from a linear, reductionist approach and toward a systems thinking approach (Craike et al., 2023). This volume attends to the complex structural challenges and inadequacies within the AMH system.

Richards et al. (2023) recommend that the need to "address gaps in the mental health system include leveraging school-based mental health programs, primary care, virtual care, and emerging models" (Richards et al., 2023). Therefore, a change across the systems that impinge on AMH is proposed here to address these complex challenges.

4.4.2 Systems Change

By definition, systems change transforms the assumptions, principles, structures, components, and processes comprising the system(s). Kania et al. (2018, p. 2) note from the Social Generation of Canada's definition of systems change as "shifting the conditions that hold the problem in place." Similarly, the World Resources Institute (2024) defines systems change as "shifting component parts of a system—and the pattern of interactions between these parts—to ultimately form a new system that behaves in a qualitatively different way."

A helpful analogy is to look at the need for systems change within the complex scope of challenges for climate change. One practical example could be the need to reduce fossil fuels in manufacturing automobiles. One area for change to achieve that goal involves the independent assembly lines making parts for electric cars. Imagine that the batteries are made in Austin, Texas, but the motor is manufactured in Shanghai, China. It takes a different system to oversee how the batteries, motors, and an estimated 22,000 other parts make their way to Fremont, California, where the electric car parts are assembled into a new Tesla (Ventura, 2023).

The same is true regarding a new approach to adolescent mental health. If independent, incremental changes are made within the "assembly lines" of the three adolescent mental health systems, and these changes are operating independently, then the root cause cannot be addressed sufficiently. A solution is to acknowledge the system boundaries and professional norms and intentionally translate knowledge formally among and between the systems. Additional shared agreements can set the parameters for communication about the best strategic, interconnected direction within each individual system and the point of intersection among the three systems.

Change, however, can be slow, as seen with climate change. Indeed, it has been 30 years since the IOM's Mental Health Continuum of Care Model was released and endorsed by the Substance Abuse and Mental Health Services Administration (SAMHSA), the primary agency in the US Department of Health and Human Services (HHS) responsible for the nation's behavioral health (IOM, 1994). Included in this mental health continuum are health promotion, prevention, early intervention, treatment, and recovery, which are essentially a "public health approach." Now this mental health continuum of care model has the possibility of being implemented. During the past few years, the AMH system, professions and scholars, including psychiatry, psychology and social work, have declared that there should be considerations for a public health approach to adolescent mental health.

Two perspectives are consistently needed to affect systems change. The first involves identifying and categorizing the macro "root causes" that contribute to the current state of poor adolescent mental health (the "crisis"). Within this framework, conducting a thorough assessment of local internal and external systems structures and processes is necessary. Each system operates within a unique sociocultural milieu with existing services and programs, some of which are quite successful in their own right. The key is to identify the intersections and iterations between the systems. Second, a microlevel analysis necessitates an understanding of the roles played by various stakeholder groups, resource opportunities, and specific community needs and limitations and their impact on the individual (Bronfenbrenner, 1979). Achieving systems change demands a purposeful connection of the global to the local in an ongoing dance that evolves with time, influenced by both successes and failures. An overburdened and inadequate AMH system can be improved and therefore help to manage the crisis.

A systems integration of public health and education systems plays a significant role with AMH (Fig. 4.1), and simple changes or programmatic fixes are not sufficient interventions. The multifactorial reasons that cause increased adverse impacts on adolescents (with potentially fewer protective effects) dictate that proposed solutions be multifactorial as well. Addressing symptoms of the problems or surface level problems has not worked. Instead, root causes must be identified and addressed, along with an analysis of the interconnected factors that perpetuate problems and inequities. Addressing the interconnections of the three core systems is one way to begin.

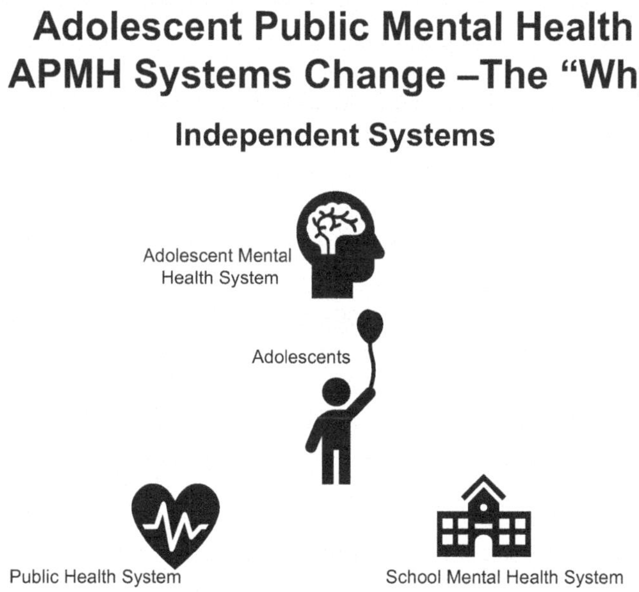

Fig. 4.1 Adolescent public mental health (APMH) systems change—the "why"

4.4.3 Convergence of Systems

With support and endorsement of a public health approach with the mental health professions, convergence among the three core AMH systems is beginning to emerge in other ways as well. Currently, there are AMH systems change ideas emerging globally and in the USA (Richards et al., 2023). Several recent publications call for a "paradigm for youth mental health" (Uhlhaas et al., 2021, 2023).

In the USA, there is movement in state legislation regarding mental health education in the schools. Texas law requires school counselors to spend at least 80% of their time providing counseling services, as opposed to conducting non-counseling duties. This time includes responsive services for students with mental health concerns (Texas Education Agency, n.d.). As per the SAVE act, New York requires school workers to receive mental health training (New York State Education Department, 2024). California, like a few other states, passed legislation requiring schools to provide mental health education. To continue the climate change comparison, California has declared that beginning in 2035, all automobiles must be electric. When there is a climate change crisis, fueled in part by fossil fuels, innovation with electric cars creates a decreased demand for gas-powered vehicles. When there is an adolescent mental health crisis, a similar, transformative systems change is required to improve mental health and well-being for adolescents, decreasing the need for treatment amid national and global shortages of providers (Fazel & Soneson, 2023).

Figure 4.2 depicts a visual convergence of the three core systems that are a part of the proposed APMH model. In the early part of the twentieth century, there was general alignment across the three developing systems. Then with the professionalization of the systems, along with a medical care system built on the biomedical model and focused on treatment, the systems became siloed. Since the latter part of the twentieth century, there has been a distinctive movement toward convergence in adolescent mental health research, practice, and the affiliated professions.

4.5 Constructing a New Adolescent Public Mental Health (APMH) Model

The proposed APMH model comprises the three systems that are now converging during the twenty-first century. Chapter 2 provided detail about adolescent mental health, and Chap. 3 provided an overview about adolescent school mental health since the latter part of the twentieth century. Therefore, this section will feature the public health approach and a relatively new term, *public mental health*.

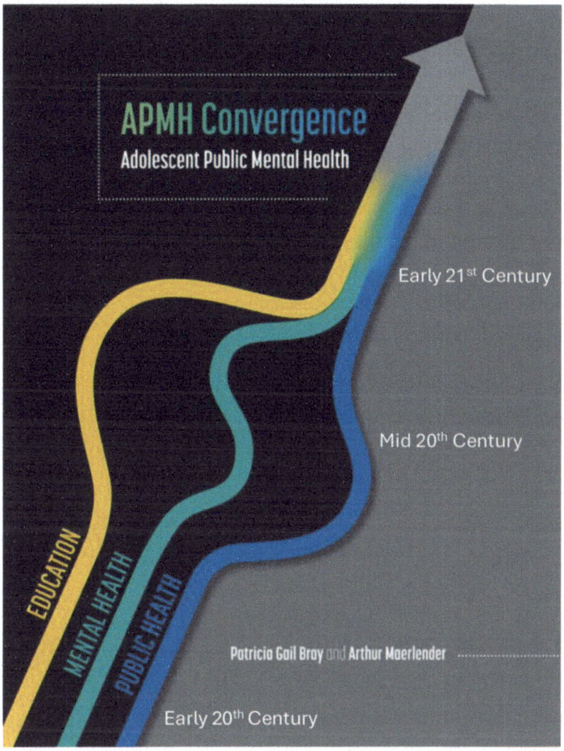

Fig. 4.2 Adolescent public mental health convergence

4.5.1 Adolescents and Public Health

Adolescent health has experienced dramatic changes during the twenty-first century. Mental health and substance abuse have become a "public health of consequence," elevating the importance for a call to action for adolescent mental health and well-being (Galea & Vaughan, 2016; Kapadia, 2024). This is a significant distinction in public health because there is recognition and acknowledgment for improvement in adolescent mental health and serves as a call to action regarding public health scholarship.

The emergence of public health efforts with adolescent mental health during the past 20 years is multifaceted, reflecting an evolving understanding of mental health and society's approach to mental well-being. Public health shares the progress seen in the adolescent mental health field due to the mental health profession's call for a public health approach to adolescent mental health (Craike et al., 2023). The key adolescent mental health milestones and developments identified in Box 4.2 are shared with public health.

Box 4.2: Adolescent Mental Health Key Milestones in the Twenty-First Century

1. Recognition of AMH as a global priority
2. Focus on resilience and social, emotional, and academic development
3. Focus on prevention and early intervention
4. Intersectional approaches with SDOH and mental health
5. Integration of mental health into schools
6. Research and evidence-based practices, including well-being
7. Research on adolescent brain development
8. Digital mental health interventions
    - Online counseling and mental health apps
    - Telehealth services
9. Trauma-informed care approaches
10. Peer support and advocacy
11. Reduction of stigma and increase in mental health literacy

4.6 APMH Themes and Goals

Given the research, the national and global declarations, and the desire to get to the root of AMH problems, broadening the scope for a new model requires an expansion beyond the absence of disease. This is especially true for a new adolescent mental health model. As mentioned earlier, the basic structure of the proposed APMH model is not really new. The IOM (1994) model justified this need by integrating a public health approach of promotion and prevention to the biomedical focus on treatment of disease. Elements of the Engel (1977) and Bronfenbrenner's (1979) expansion of the biomedical model were included in the IOM model, which helps to justify the applicability of the model to adolescent mental health.

The APMH model uses that same basic structure with enhanced features. These include a recognition of the core system interconnections that play a role in the unique developmental changes that occur in adolescence. The APMH model also integrates the nonmedical factors—the social determinants of health—with intentional acknowledgment about the role these factors play in adolescent growth and development. The research is conclusive that growing up in poverty has significant implications for educational inequities, causing poor health, including poor mental health (Gorski & Landsman, 2014).

During the twenty-first century, the scholarship and needed subsequent action regarding equity have evolved to become an embedded part of health improvement. Therefore, the APMH model embeds the idea of systems integration and equity as the two primary themes, resulting in two goals:

1. The first goal is to develop an AMH model that represents the proposed systems change of integrating AMH with public health and school health. This model

streamlines four evidence-based frameworks, including mental health literacy (social emotional learning or SEL), a multitiered system of supports (MTSS), which are discussed in the School Health chapter. Additionally, the social determinants of health (SDOH) are integrated into the APMH model and will be discussed in a later section. Finally, a multisector, collaborative approach called collective impact (CI) is a key component to the model and is discussed in the Strategies chapter.
2. The second goal is to share an APMH implementation approach encompassing the four frameworks (SEL, MTSS, SDOH, and CI) that can be adopted and adapted within any culture and environment throughout the world. Additionally, the model should be nimble enough to incorporate new research methodologies and policies, such as with adolescents and social media.

4.7 APMH Five Principles

This new, proposed universal APMH model augments the existing AMH system by emphasizing five key principles that are outlined and woven throughout the chapters in this volume and are included in Table 4.1. All of the principles operate on the premise of embedded notions of integration and equity.

Table 4.1 Adolescent public mental health—APMH five principles

APMH model—five principles	APMH model integration approaches
Principle 1 Adopt the Social Ecological Model	Prioritize an expanded version of the biomedical model to include the biopsychosocial model and the social determinants of health, culminating in a social ecological model
Principle 2 Implement Strategies for Population and Individual Levels of Health	Implement strategies that address the broader population while also promoting health, and prevention and early intervention of mental disorders for individual adolescents
Principle 3 Acknowledge the Whole Child/Adolescent	Acknowledge the interconnectedness of adolescent physical, mental, social, and emotional well-being, by addressing all aspects holistically; acknowledge the connections between individuals, families, school, the social, and community
Principle 4 Foster Multisector Collaboration in Schools	Foster multisector collaboration in schools, including education, healthcare, community organizations, and families, to support adolescent mental health and well-being within the school environment
Principle 5 Create a New Model based on a "Public Mental Health Approach" in Schools	Create and implement a new school-based model based on the intersections of public health, mental health, and education. Prioritize an equitable, holistic adolescent mental system with health promotion and mental disorder prevention, early intervention, and the social determinants of health

4.7.1 Principle 1: Adopt the Social Ecological Model

The first principle acknowledges the hallmark of the biomedical model, which is that the absence of disease defines health and well-being. However, this narrow view of health has expanded during the past 50 years to embrace the biopsychosocial aspects of health (Engel, 1977), Bronfenbrenner's ecological systems theory (Bronfenbrenner, 1979) and the social determinants of health, and the nonmedical factors that influence health and well-being (Marmot & Wilkinson, 1999). The social ecological model, therefore, includes this expanded meaning of health, which closely aligns with the WHO's definition of health (1948) and is considered a framework for prevention (CDC, n.d.). CDC asserts that the social ecological model "considers the complex interplay between individual, relationship, community, and societal factors." There is general consensus that this expanded view of health and well-being represents the "wide-ranging manifestations of youth." Due to the significant developments during adolescence, it is noted that they are particularly impacted by the environmental context (Uhlhaas et al., 2023).

Therefore, the social determinants of health help to round out this first principle. Following the research regarding the social ecological model, important milestones were reached with the development and acceptance of the social determinants of health—those nonmedical factors that are inextricably tied to health and well-being. The realization of the impacts of social, economic, and environmental factors that impinge on individual health marked a profound shift in thinking about health (including mental health). This work opened up the discussion in public health, which extended the definition of health to include the effects of the social and physical environment and genetics on well-being and prosperity.

A seminal article on the SDOH was published in 1990 by the Canadian Institute for Advanced Research scholars, Evans and Stoddart. Their insight featured a bold thesis that asserted that the impacts of nonmedical factors directly and indirectly affect the individual's physical health. This in turn allowed the focus of treatment to move beyond treating only the individual. See Box 4.3 for the WHO's recent, partial list of the SDOH (WHO, 2024).

Box 4.3: Nonmedical Factors for Health: Social Determinants of Health from the WHO (2024)

- Income and social protection
- Education
- Access to quality, affordable health services
- Early childhood development
- Social inclusion and nondiscrimination
- Housing, basic amenities, and the environment
- Food insecurity
- Working life conditions
- Unemployment and job insecurity
- Structural conflict

Poor adolescent health and well-being are not caused by disease alone. There are also social, cultural, and societal challenges that contribute to adolescent mental health challenges. Evans and Stoddart (1990) proposed that the healthcare system and genetics accounted for about 20% of our health. The significant impacts on our health, they argued, came from the environment and social interactions, including behavioral aspects, accounting for about 80% of health.

Initially, the SDOH referred to the physcial aspects of health. However, the social determinants of mental health (SDOMH) are now recognized nonmedical factors that disrupt optimal health and increase risk for physical *and* mental illness (Compton & Shim, 2015). The SDOH are defined by the WHO (2024) as:

> The nonmedical factors that influence health outcomes. They are the conditions in which people are born, grow, work, live, and age, and the wider set of forces and systems shaping the conditions of daily life. These forces and systems include economic policies and systems, development agendas, social norms, social policies, racism, climate change and political systems.

The SDOH serve an important and vital role regarding health equities (Marmot & Wilkinson, 1999; WHO, 2024) During the late 1990s, researchers at University College London partnered with the World Health Organization to draft a groundbreaking publication called the *Social Determinants of Health—The Solid Facts* (Wilkinson & Marmot, 1998). This research was fundamental to the *Independent Inquiry into Inequalities in Health*, a report commissioned by the UK government the same year (Acheson, 1998; cited in Marmot & Wilkinson, 1999), thus beginning a transformative change to public health, globally, and in the USA. By including nonmedical factors in a more just and equitable approach to the understanding of health outcomes, the move beyond an exclusively biomedical model had begun. This transformative shift has helped to shape science, policy, and practice during the twenty-first century.

The adoption of the SDOH has been a slow process, unfolding during the past four and one-half decades (Osmick & Wilson, 2020). In 2020, the WHO published *Conceptual Framework for Action on the Social Determinants of Health* (2010) that has significantly affected social and public policies by pushing for inclusion of health equity in community programs and educational training. Now, research supporting health equity has been integrated with both public health and mental health education systems. The importance of this shift cannot be overstated as the empirical support has lent credibility to acknowledging the interconnections of poverty, environmental degradation, and inequality with health and well-being.

4.7.2 Principle 2: Implement Strategies for Population and Individual Levels of Health

The second key principle also represents an integration between public health and medicine. By adopting the social ecological model, adolescent mental health solutions by definition operate at a population level *and* an individual level. Population health is a key feature in public health defined as more than one individual, sharing one or more common characteristics (Shultz et al., 2021, p. 3). Systems change necessarily operates at a population level, since system policies, guidelines, and protocols determine how to promote population health *and* prevent and treat illness for individual patients. Promoting health and preventing disease have always been a core function of public health, defined as "the science and art of preventing disease, prolonging life, and promoting health through the organized efforts and informed choices of society, organizations, public and private communities, and individuals" (Winslow, 1920). Since the mid-twentieth century, medicine was largely dominated by the biomedical model, which emphasized the role of biological processes and pathological mechanisms in disease causation and treatment. Physicians adhered to the biomedical model primarily focused on diagnosing diseases based on signs, symptoms, and laboratory tests and treating them with pharmaceuticals, surgery, or other medical interventions. A convergence in public health and medicine could change the AMH system to be more compatible.

4.7.2.1 Public Health and Medicine

One could surmise that during the 1940s, with Paul Lemkau's (1949) vision of integrated public health and mental health systems and the WHO's (1948) holistic definition of health, we were poised for an integrated, holistic health system in both public health and medicine. Mental health was not yet separated arbitrarily from physical health. A person's well-being is not possible if their mental health is challenged, for example, with major depressive disorder. Likewise, a person cannot experience well-being, including mental well-being, if they are sick with a 103-degree fever caused by influenza.

Adopting an adolescent public health approach creates an integration between public health and medicine generally at several levels. Emphasizing prevention *and* treatment leads to more holistic treatment that gives equal importance to mind and body at the individual level and the population health level. Additionally, by including nonmedical factors, or social determinants of health, the mental and physical risk factors are broadened, allowing for a better understanding of appropriate interventions. This in turn affects research, policy, and advocacy for more culturally sensitive and equitable responses for population health.

4.7.3 Principle 3: Acknowledge the Whole Child/Adolescent

The third principle represents an integration of the physical, mental, and social well-being aspects of an adolescent, following the World Health Organization's (1948) definition of health. Adolescent physical, mental, and social health are not independent states but exist in mutually supporting processes. The Centers for Disease

Control and Prevention (CDC, 2014) created a *Whole School, Whole Community, and Whole Child* (WSCC) model that formalizes the interdependent nature with 10 components, including the schools, community, families, and students. During the twenty-first century, there has been incremental movement to see the *whole* child and adolescent.

4.7.3.1 CDC Whole School, Whole Community, Whole Child Model

The USA Centers for Disease Control and Prevention has a long history of strongly advocating for school-based health initiatives. Their justification scientifically reinforces the fact that healthy, "whole" students leads to more effective learning. Copious research shows academic achievement helps to ensure a future of lifetime successes. Together in 2014, with the Association for Supervision and Curriculum Development (ASCD), CDC developed the Whole School, Whole Community, Whole Child (WSCC) model (CDC, 2014). The WSCC introduced important components to a student-centered approach with the realization that the child is influenced by and engaged with their families, schools, and communities, as well as the policies and processes that affect the life of the child/adolescent.

The premise is that "every child in every school deserves to be a healthy, safe, engaged, supported and challenged" (CDC, 2018). This community model shows that by coordinating policy, process, and practice, with a whole school, community, and child approach, learning and health are improved. The components are listed in Box 4.4.

When this model was developed, there was a recognition that alignment of education, public health, and school health was critical to success. Families, schools, and communities are intertwined within the theoretical concepts of the WSCC model in order to work together to nurture the health and education of the whole child. The first 8 of the 10 WSCC components (with the asterisk) align with the APMH model.

Box 4.4: CDC Components to WSCC Model (CDC, 2018)

Counseling, psychological, and social services*
Social and emotional climate*
Family engagement*
Community involvement*
Physical education and activity*
Physical environment*
Health education*
Health services*
Nutrition environment and services
Employee wellness

4.7.4 Principle 4: Foster Multisector Collaboration in Schools

The fourth principle is to create a multisector collaboration with various sectors in the community who can become partners in the implementation of the new model. Initiating strategic systems change that directly fosters effective collaboration for the prevention and treatment of adolescent mental ill-health is an ambitious goal. Achieving this objective demands the meticulous crafting of a multisector commitment and concerted action, within a collaborative framework, such as collective impact (Kania & Kramer, 2011). The approach recommended here for the adolescent public mental health collaboration framework has proven effective for the implementation of complex, intractable problems, such as the ongoing AMH challenges (Counts et al., 2018).

4.7.5 Principle 5: Create a Public Health Approach

Principle 5 asserts that current adolescent mental healthcare in the USA is in actuality "mental sickness care" (Insel, 2022, p. xxiii). Instead of focusing on illness, adopting the IOM public health approach is a critical pivot. Waiting for adolescent problems to emerge in the form of psychiatric disorders and behavioral disruptions is the approach of traditional mental healthcare. Building mental health literacy and practicing prevention in schools help identify mental health disorders earlier, with shorter treatment time. Integrating the social determinants of health helps to address equity by identifying nonmedical factors that affect mental health. The integration and alignment of the core systems places the adolescent at the center of a new APMH model.

4.8 A Note on *Public Mental Health*

A public health approach is a broad framework that applies public health concepts, such as promotion, prevention, and social determinants to a specific concern and is not limited to mental health. *A public mental health* approach specifically aligns public health with mental health. Dykxhoorn et al. (2022) define public mental health as "the science and art of promoting mental health and well-being and preventing mental health problems through organised efforts of society" (citing Acheson, 1988).

The mental health literature speaks of a "public health approach" and "public mental health," with both concepts sharing a population health focus. By integrating existing individual level approaches with population health level approaches, it becomes feasible to provide systems that inform and normalize the standards of healthy environments, destigmatize mental healthcare, and, in the case of AMH, provide earlier treatment to the individual adolescent.

A public mental health approach "requires the study and monitoring of which diseases and disorders are present in the population" (Eaton & Fallin, 2019, p. xv). Additionally, a public mental health approach includes population-based strategies for "collective or social actions" (Fazel & Soneson, 2023, quoting Last, 2001, p. 145) and an emphasis on prevention over treatment, among other considerations that broaden the mental health purview outside of traditional health settings" (See for example, Campion, 2018; Eaton & Fallin, 2019; Fazel & Soneson, 2023). The result is a more holistic understanding of mental health in schools and communities, although it has taken many decades to arrive here.

A 1948 article in the *Canadian Journal of Public Health* discussed an integrated public mental health concept by joining mental hygiene concepts with public health practices (Schumacher, 1948). Fifteen years later, more attention to aspects of public mental health indirectly impacted the passage of the 1963 USA Community Mental Health Act, which focused on providing care to adults with intellectual and developmental disabilities in community-based settings rather than institutions.

There is evidence that public mental health research began to gain traction during the 1980s (Wahlbeck, 2015, p. 38). During the end of the twentieth century and especially since the beginning of the twenty-first century, there has been more attention to the concept of public mental health. The interconnection in the shared space between the two fields of public health and mental health is part of the basis for *public mental health*.

The *American Journal of Public Health* celebrated its 75th anniversary in 1985. One of the review articles, *Public Health Aspects of Mental Health: The last 75 years of the American Journal of Public Health*, noted that "early authors on public mental health lobbied strongly for the inclusion of mental health in the field of public health" (Williams & Westermeyer, 1985, p. 723). This statement harkens back to the early days of public health and mental health, which affirmed the importance of including mental health with public health, as well the fact that public health is vital to the field of mental health, as observed with the formation of the first School of Public Health at Johns Hopkins in 1916 (Johns Hopkins Bloomberg School of Public Health (n.d.)).

In 1996, the WHO released a document that foreshadowed public mental health today, titled "Public Mental Health: Guidelines for the Elaboration and Management of National Mental Health Programmes" (World Health Organization, 1997). Surprisingly, despite offering specific definitions for various mental health aspects, and the implicit integration of mental health with public health, the document does not provide a definition for the term "public mental health."

During the twenty-first century, we see a marked increase globally, especially in the UK, of attention to the concept of public mental health and the move to integrate public health and mental health. Fears and Höschl (2011) published an opinion piece in the *European Journal of Public Health*, "European Mental Health Policy Should Target Everybody." This was followed a few years later with a recommendation to translate public mental health evidence into practice, motivated by the assertion that "public mental health is coming of age and is increasingly being accepted as an important and integral part of both public health and mental health" (Wahlbeck, 2015, p. 40).

Eaton and Fallin (2019) agree with this assertion, as they note in their groundbreaking book, *Public Mental Health*, that the focus on public mental health has accelerated. They articulate the conceptual basis for "the public health approach to mental and behavioral disorders," which is adopted in this volume. The intent of this volume is to build on their work by applying a public mental health approach to the adolescent population, specifically.

4.9 The Promise of an Adolescent Public Mental Health Model

The public mental health principles, systems, and concepts forms the basis of the adolescent public mental health (APMH) school-based model that represents a transformative systems change. APMH is based on the case study that describes the 7-year, foundation grant-funded project developed and implemented in the Greater Houston, Texas, region. The case study required SEL, MTSS and multisector collaboration to be implemented with the collective impact (CI) strategy, which included secondary schools and community agencies, including for profit and non-profit mental health providers, such as The Menninger Clinic. The learnings from the implementation of the project became the model for the proposed integrations described here and offers important lessons informed by science. The next step involves moving the APMH model into the mainstream of professions, policies, and practice, in order to further research in the AMH field.

The COVID-19 pandemic has increased the urgency and momentum that has been growing globally regarding the increased adolescent mental health problems. The driving question is how best to design, develop, and implement the model nationally and globally? *Adolescent public mental health* is a new term that has recently emerged in the scientific literature (Fazel & Soneson, 2023). The proposed APMH model in this volume is a construct that includes the three interconnected core systems. Each of the systems contains an independent and interdependent historical context along with a depth and breadth of knowledge, which is reviewed in more detail in a later chapter. The outcome is the introduction of this new, advanced adolescent public mental health model (Fig. 4.3), designed for implementation in schools. Although the process encompasses numerous inherent complexities, it can be analogous to other complex systems theories, such as climate change, with the interconnections and need for adaptation and resilience.

4.10 Conclusion

Adolescent mental health has experienced significant shifts during the twenty-first century. At its core, the proposed APMH model underscores collaboration and seeks to enhance the mental health and well-being of students by adopting a public mental

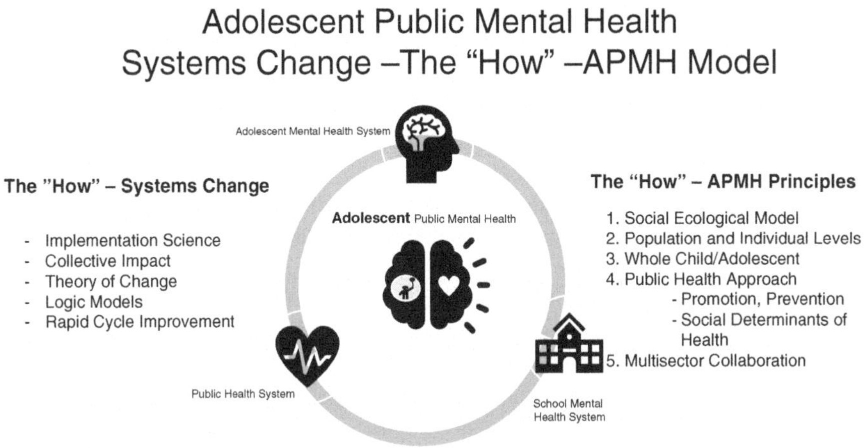

Fig. 4.3 Adolescent public mental health systems change—the "how"—APMH model

health approach. In this context, public health embraces both the biopsychosocial framework and the social ecological model, integrating evidence-based approaches for the whole child, addressing both mental and physical health, and encompassing schools, families, and communities. The relationship between public health, mental health, and school health has become increasingly interconnected, recognizing the importance of a holistic approach and systems change to address the well-being of adolescents. These comprehensive approaches reflect the essence of the mental "hygiene" movement (later known as the mental health movement) in the USA. During this earlier movement, intentional synergy between mental health and public health emerged, foreshadowing the state of the research currently. These arguments include advocating for a holistic view, recognizing the significance of prevention and collaboration, and understanding that social and environmental factors profoundly impact mental health.

Like climate change, transforming adolescent public mental health involves addressing complex challenges and requires systems change. Local, regional, state, national, and international leaders can help to create policies, mandates, and guidelines that will encourage APMH to be implemented in every school. And, like climate change, the exponential acceleration of the problems associated with APMH call for decisive and bold changes which can stem the aggressive rise of concerns. A multisector approach to mental health prevention and early intervention for all adolescents in every secondary school represents an innovative, integrated solution.

So, what happened? What happened to cause the chasm between mental health and physical health in medicine and, in part, in public health? Why was mental health marginalized from both? And why is now an optimal time for a systems change in adolescent public mental health?

1. Medicine adopted the biomedical model, which led to a focus on diseases and treatment.
2. The focus on disease led to a proliferation of medical specialty areas, creating silos of health.
3. In part due to technology, the healthcare system was preoccupied with curing disease and not overall well-being.
4. If medical professionals could not identify a disease process with a microscope, then it was marginalized and excluded. This caused a stigma around mental health.
5. Although mental health and social health were part of the WHO definition of health, psychiatry endured a disadvantage with a biomedical model that did not include mental health factors of health.
6. Although WHO's definition included a state of complete physical, mental, and social well-being, the next 50 years embraced a healthcare system structure focused on treatment aspects for physical disorders.
7. The poverty and educational factors, along with other nonmedical determinants of health, such as housing, were excluded from the biomedical model for similar reasons as the mental ones.
8. The fragmentation of services precluded a holistic approach to health.

During the twenty-first century, we have evolved scientifically to a more integrated notion of physical, mental, and social factors affecting well-being. The policies, professional guidelines and practices slowly converge with the scientific shift. Big systems typically change slowly, especially within a sector as large as healthcare. What has been occurring in the last 5–10 years addresses some of these structures that are institutionally entrenched and are now showing signs of a positive shift. Along with institutional old "ways of life," there are also cultural and societal biases toward how "things have always been done this way." That said, there is recent cause of optimism with moving ever closer to that 75-year-old WHO (1948) definition of health that includes the following:

- Promote preventive measures—holistically
- Integrate mental health with public health and primary care
- Address social determinants of health
- Address racial and ethnic bias as determinants of health
- Engage in multisector collaboration

The National Research Council and Institute of Medicine (2009) noted that the USA is well positioned to help young people live happier and healthier lives and that it "can be achieved by refining the science and by developing the infrastructure and large-scale collaborative systems that allow the equitable delivery of population-based preventive approaches." Their optimism can possibly come to fruition in the near future.

Competing Interests *The authors have no conflicts of interest to declare that are relevant to the content of this chapter.*

Further Reading

Alegria, M., Alvarez, K., Cheng, M., & Falgas-Bague, I. (2023, July 1). Recent advances on social determinants of mental health: Looking fast forward. *The American Journal of Psychiatry*. https://doi.org/10.1176/appi.ajp.20230371

Backes, E. P., Bonnie, R. J., & National Academies of Sciences, Engineering, and Medicine, Division of Behavioral and Social Sciences and Education, Health and Medicine Division, Board on Children, Youth, and Families, & Committee on the Neurobiological and Socio-behavioral Science of Adolescent Development and Its Applications. (2019). *The promise of adolescence*. National Academies Press eBooks. The National Academies Press. https://doi.org/10.17226/25388

Bauman, A. (2022, November 17). Texas children's ER sees massive spike in kids with mental health crises like suicidal thoughts. *Houston Chronicle* Retrieved March 19, 2024, from http://www.houstonchronicle.com/news/houston-texas/health/article/Texas-Childrens-Hospital-ER-visits-17589153.php

Braveman, P., Egerter, S., & Williams, D. R. (2011). The social determinants of health: Coming of age. *Annual Review of Public Health, 32*, 381–398. https://doi.org/10.1146/annurev-publhealth-031210-101218

Breuner, C. C., & Bell, D. L. (2023). Adolescent mental and behavioral health: COVID-19 exacerbation of a prevailing crisis. *Pediatrics, 151*(Supplement 1). https://doi.org/10.1542/peds.2022-057267d

Centers for Disease Control and Prevention. (2020a). *Healthy people 2030*. Healthcare access and quality. Retrieved April 19, 2024, from https://health.gov/healthypeople/objectives-and-data/browse-objectives/health-care-access-and-quality

Centers for Disease Control and Prevention. (2020b). *Healthy people 2030*. Education access. Retrieved April 19, 2024, from https://health.gov/healthypeople/objectives-and-data/browse-objectives/education-access-and-quality

Centers for Disease Control and Prevention. (2020c). *Healthy people 2030*. Social and community context. Retrieved April 19, 2024, from https://health.gov/healthypeople/objectives-and-data/browse-objectives/social-and-community-context.

Centers for Disease Control and Prevention. (2020d). *Healthy people 2030*. Neighborhood and built environment. Retrieved April 19, 2024, from https://health.gov/healthypeople/objectives-and-data/browse-objectives/neighborhood-and-built-environment

Centers for Disease Control and Prevention. (2020e). *Healthy people 2030*. Economic stability. Retrieved April 19, 2024, from https://health.gov/healthypeople/objectives-and-data/browse-objectives/economic-stability

Centers for Disease Control and Prevention. (2020f). *Healthy people 2030*. What are the social determinants of health? Retrieved April 30, 2024, from https://health.gov/healthypeople/priority-areas/social-determinants-health

Detrow, S. (2021, October 19). Kids' mental health crisis is at a critical point, education secretary Cardona says. *NPR Morning Edition*. Education Interview.

Hafstad, G. S., Sætren, S. S., Wentzel-Larsen, T., & Augusti, E. M. (2021). Adolescents' symptoms of anxiety and depression before and during the COVID-19 outbreak—A prospective population-based study of teenagers in Norway. *The Lancet Regional Health, 2021*. https://doi.org/10.1016/j.lanepe.2021.100093

Hoge, M. A., Vanderploeg, J., Paris, M., Jr., Lang, J. M., & Olezeski, C. (2022). Emergency department use by children and youth with mental health conditions: A health equity agenda. *Community Mental Health Journal, 58*(7), 1225–1239. https://doi.org/10.1007/s10597-022-00937-7

Johns, M. M., Lowry, R., Haderxhanaj, L. T., Rasberry, C. N., Robin, L., Scales, L., Stone, D., & Suarez, N. A. (2020). Trends in violence victimization and suicide risk by sexual identity among high school students – Youth risk behavior survey. United States, 2015–2019. *MMWR Supplements, 69*(1), 19–27. https://doi.org/10.15585/mmwr.su6901a3

Kalb, L. G., Stapp, E. K., Ballard, E. D., Holingue, C., Keefer, A., & Riley, A. (2019). Trends in psychiatric emergency department visits among youth and young adults in the US. *Pediatrics, 143*, 4.e20182192. https://doi.org/10.1542/peds.2018-2192

Kania, J., Williams, J., Schmitz, P., Brady, S., Kramer, M., & Juster, J. S. (2022, Winter). Centering equity in collective impact. *Stanford Social Innovation Review*. Retrieved February 7, 2024, from https://ssir.org/articles/entry/centering_equity_in_collective_impact

Kessler, R. C., Amminger, G. P., Aguilar-Gaxiola, S., Alonso, J., Lee, P., & Üstün, T. B. (2007). Age of onset of mental disorders: A review of recent literature. *Current Opinion in Psychiatry, 20*(4), 359–364. https://doi.org/10.1097/yco.0b013e32816ebc8c

Murthy, V. H. (2023). *Our epidemic of loneliness and isolation. The U.S. Surgeon General's Advisory*. U.S. Department of Health and Human Services Retrieved March 31, 2024, from https://www.hhs.gov/sites/default/files/surgeon-general-social-connection-advisory.pdf

Piao, J., Huang, Y., Han, C., et al. (2022). Alarming changes in the global burden of mental disorders in children and adolescents from 1990 to 2019: A systematic analysis for the global burden of disease study. *European Child & Adolescent Psychiatry, 31*, 1827–1845. https://doi.org/10.1007/s00787-022-02040-4

Shim, R. S., & Compton, M. T. (2020). The social determinants of mental health: Psychiatrists' roles in addressing discrimination and food insecurity. *Focus (American Psychiatric Publishing), 18*(1), 25–30. https://doi.org/10.1176/appi.focus.20190035

Substance Abuse and Mental Health Services Administration, Center for Mental Health Services. (2022). *National guidelines for child and youth behavioral health crisis care*. Retrieved September 6, 2024, from https://store.samhsa.gov/product/national-guidelines-child-and-youth-behavioral-health-crisis-care/pep22-01-02-001

Tulchinsky, T. H., & Varavikova, E. A. (2014). A history of public health. *The New Public Health*, 1–42. https://doi.org/10.1016/B978-0-12-415766-8.00001-X

Ullman, C. A. (1949, December 30). A public health approach to improving community mental health through schools. *Public Health Reports, 64*(52). Retrieved March 3, 2024, from https://www.ncbi.nlm.nih.gov/pmc/articles/PMC1997008/pdf/pubhealthreporig01240-0001.pdf

Velez, G., et al. (2022). *Social determinants of mental health in children and youth*. APA Resource Document. Approved by the Joint Reference Committee. American Psychiatric Association. Retrieved February 29, 2024, from https://www.psychiatry.org/getattachment/a03e07c5-bba9-4ac7-b434-9183b1e0b730/Resource-Document-Social-Determinants-of-Mental-Health-Youth.pdf

Weist, M. D., Hoover, S. A., Daly, B. P., Short, K. H., & Bruns, E. J. (2023). Propelling the global advancement of school mental health. *Clinical Child and Family Psychology Review, 26*(4), 851–864. https://doi.org/10.1007/s10567-023-00434-7

World Health Organization. (2001). *Strengthening mental health promotion programmes*. World Health Organization (Fact sheet, No. 220). https://www.who.int/europe/activities/strengthening-mental-health-promotion-programmes

References

Acheson, E. D. (1988). On the state of the public health [the fourth Duncan lecture]. *Public Health, 102*(5), 431–437.

Acheson, D. (1998). *Independent inquiry into health inequalities report*. The Stationery Office.

Agency for Healthcare Research and Quality. (AHRQ) (2022, October). *2022 National healthcare quality and disparities report*. Pub. No. 22(23)-0030. Retrieved March 25, 2024, from https://www.ahrq.gov/research/findings/nhqrdr/nhqdr22/index.html

American Academy of Child & Adolescent Psychiatry. (n.d.). *AACAP history*. Retrieved March 5, 2024, from https://www.aacap.org/AACAP/About_AACAP/AACAP_History.aspx

American Academy of Pediatrics. (2022, October 13). *Health organizations urge the Biden administration to declare a federal national emergency in children's mental health*. Retrieved March 27, 2024, from https://www.aap.org/en/news-room/news-releases/aap/2022/health-organizations-urge-the-biden-administration-to-declare-a-federal-national-emergency-in-childrens-mental-health/

American Academy of Pediatrics. (2024). *The birth of the AAP (1930–1949)*. Retrieved April 17, 2024, from https://www.aap.org/en/about-the-aap/gartner-pediatric-history-center/celebrating-90-years-of-adolescent-health/

American Academy of Pediatrics, American Academy of Child and Adolescent Psychiatry, & The Children's Hospital Association. (2021). *Declaration of a National Emergency in Child and Adolescent Mental Health*. https://www.aap.org/en/advocacy/child-and-adolescent-healthy-mental-development/aap-aacap-cha-declaration-of-a-national-emergency-in-child-and-adolescent-mental-health/

Bauer, M. S., & Kirchner, J. (2020). Implementation science: What is it and why should I care? *Psychiatry Research, 283*, 112376. https://doi.org/10.1016/j.psychres.2019.04.025

Bronfenbrenner, U. (1979). *The ecology of human development: Experiments by nature and design*. Harvard University Press.

Campion, J. (2018). Public mental health: Key challenges and opportunities. *BJPsych International, 3*, 51–54. Retrieved August 29, 2023, from https://www.ncbi.nlm.nih.gov/pmc/articles/PMC6690256/

Campisi, S. C., Carducci, B., Akseer, N., et al. (2020). Suicidal behaviours among adolescents from 90 countries: A pooled analysis of the global school-based student health survey. *BMC Public Health, 20*, 1102. https://doi.org/10.1186/s12889-020-09209-z

Centers for Disease Control and Prevention. (2014). *Whole school, whole community, whole child (WSCC)*. Retrieved February 28, 2023, from https://www.cdc.gov/healthyschools/wscc/index.htm

Centers for Disease Control and Prevention. (2018). *Whole school, whole community, whole child (WSCC)*. Retrieved April 10, 2023, from https://www.cdc.gov/healthyyouth/wscc/model.htm

Centers for Disease Control and Prevention. (2021). *WISQARS leading causes of death visualization tool*. Retrieved March 28, 2024, from https://wisqars.cdc.gov/lcd/?o=LCD&y1=2021&y2=2021&ct=12&cc=ALL&g=00&s=0&r=0&ry=0&e=0&ar=lcd1age&at=groups&ag=lcd1age&a1=0&a2=199

Centers for Disease Control and Prevention. (n.d.). *The social-ecological model: A framework for prevention*. Retrieved March 19, 2024, from https://www.cdc.gov/violenceprevention/about/social-ecologicalmodel.html

Compton, M. T., & Shim, R. S. (Eds.). (2015). *The social determinants of mental health*. American Psychiatric Association.

Counts, J., Gillam, R., Garstka, T. A., & Urbach, E. (2018). How the Center for Public Partnerships and Research navigates complex social problems to make a collective difference. *Journal of Evidence-Informed Social Work, 15*(3), 313–323. https://doi.org/10.1080/23761407.2018.1449158

Craike, M., Klepac, B., Mowle, A., & Riley, T. (2023). Theory of systems change: An initial, middle-range theory of public health research impact. *Research Evaluation, 32*(3), 603–621. https://doi.org/10.1093/reseval/rvad030

Curtin, S. C., & Garnett, M. F. (2023, June). *Suicide and homicide death rates among youth and young adults aged 10–24: United States, 2001–2021*. National Center for Health Statistics (NCHS). Data brief. U.S. Department of Health and Human Services. Centers for Disease Control and Prevention. Retrieved February 5, 2024, from https://www.cdc.gov/nchs/data/databriefs/db471.pdf

Dykxhoorn, J., Fischer, L., Bayliss, B., et al. (2022). Conceptualising public mental health: Development of a conceptual framework for public mental health. *BMC Public Health, 22*(1), 1407. https://doi.org/10.1186/s12889-022-13775-9

Eaton, W. W., & Fallin, D. M. (2019). *Public mental health* (2nd ed.). Oxford Unviersity Press.

Ehlman, D. C., Yard, E. E., Stone, D. M., Jones, C. M., & Mack, K. A. (2022). Changes in suicide rates—United States, 2019 and 2020. *Morbidity and Mortality Weekly Report, 71*(8), 306–312. https://doi.org/10.15585/mmwr.mm7108a5

Engel, G. L. (1977). The need for a new medical model: A challenge for biomedicine. *Science, 196*(4286), 129–136. https://doi.org/10.1126/science.847460

Erskine, H. E., Moffitt, T. E., Copeland, W. E., Costello, E. J., Ferrari, A. J., Patton, G., Degenhardt, L., Vos, T., Whiteford, H. A., & Scott, J. G. (2015). A heavy burden on young minds: The global burden of mental and substance use disorders in children and youth. *Psychological Medicine, 45*(7), 1551–1563. https://doi.org/10.1017/S0033291714002888

Evans, R. G., & Stoddart, G. L. (1990). Producing health, consuming health care. *Social Science & Medicine, 31*(12), 1347–1363. Accessed April 11, 2023, from. https://doi.org/10.1016/0277-9536(90)90074-3

Fazel, M., & Soneson, E. (2023). Current evidence and opportunities in child and adolescent public mental health: A research review. *Journal of Child Psychology and Psychiatry, 64*(12), 1699–1719. https://doi.org/10.1111/jcpp.13889

Fears, R., & Höschl, C. (2011). European mental health policy: Opportunities for science and innovation, challenges for implementation. *European Journal of Public Health, 21*(5), 550–551. https://doi.org/10.1093/eurpub/ckr075

Galea, S., & Vaughan, R. (2016). A public health of consequence. *American Journal of Public Health, 106*(1), 10–11. https://doi.org/10.2105/AJPH.2015.302954

García-Fernández, L., Romero-Ferreiro, V., Izquierdo-Izquierdo, M., Rodriguez, V. N., Álvarez-Mon, M. Á., Lahera, G., Santos, J. L., & Rodríguez-Jiménez, R. (2023). Dramatic increase of suicidality in children and adolescents after COVID-19 pandemic start: A two-year longitudinal study. *Journal of Psychiatric Research, 163*, 63–67. https://doi.org/10.1016/j.jpsychires.2023.04.014

Gorski, P. C., & Landsman, J. (2014). *The poverty and education reader: A call for equity in many voices* (1st ed.). Routledge. https://www.routledge.com/The-Poverty-and-Education-Reader-A-Call-for-Equity-in-Many-Voices/Gorski-Landsman/p/book/9781579228590

Gramlich, J. (2023a). *Gun deaths among U.S. children and teens rose 50% in two years*. Pew Research Center. Retrieved March 28, 2024, from https://www.pewresearch.org/short-reads/2023/04/06/gun-deaths-among-us-kids-rose-50-percent-in-two-years/

Gramlich, J. (2023b). *What the data says about gun deaths in the U.S.* Pew Research Center. Retrieved March 31, 2024, from https://www.pewresearch.org/short-reads/2023/04/26/what-the-data-says-about-gun-deaths-in-the-u-s/

Hall, G. S. (1904). *Adolescence its psychology and its relations to physiology, anthropology, sociology sex, crime, religion and education, Vol. II*. Appleton. https://doi.org/10.1037/10618-000

Healy, W. (1915). *The individual delinquent: A text-book of diagnosis and prognosis for all concerned in understanding offenders*. Little, Brown.

Hurst, A., Shaw, N., Carrieri, D., Stein, K., & Wyatt, K. (2024). Exploring the rise and diversity of health and societal issues that use a public health approach: A scoping review and narrative synthesis. *PLOS Global Public Health, 4*(1), e0002790. https://doi.org/10.1371/journal.pgph.0002790

Insel, T. (2022). *Healing: Our path from mental illness to mental health*. Penguin Press.

Institute of Medicine. (1994). *Reducing risks for mental disorder: Frontiers for preventive intervention research* (P. J. Mrazek & R. J. Haggerty, Eds.). National Academy of Sciences.

Johns Hopkins Bloomberg School of Public Health. (n.d.). *History*. Retrieved February 29, 2024, https://publichealth.jhu.edu/about/history

Jones, E. A. K., Mitra, A. K., & Bhuiyan, A. R. (2021). Impact of COVID-19 on mental health in adolescents: A systematic review. *International Journal of Environmental Research and Public Health, 18*(5), 2470. https://doi.org/10.3390/ijerph18052470

Kania, J., & Kramer, M. (2011). Collective impact. *Stanford Social Innovation Review*. https://ssir.org/articles/entry/collective_impact

Kania, J., Kramer, M., & Senge, P. (2018). The water of systems change. *FSG: Reimagining Social Change*. Retrieved February 5, 2024, from https://www.fsg.org/wp-content/uploads/2021/08/The-Water-of-Systems-Change_rc.pdf

Kapadia, F. (2024). Adolescent mental health and well-being: A public health of consequence, February 2024. *American Journal of Public Health, 114*(2), 158–160. https://doi.org/10.2105/AJPH.2023.307543

Kaufman Family Foundation (KFF). (2023). *News release. U.S. has the highest rate of gun deaths for children and teens among peer countries*. Retrieved March 28, 2024, from https://www.kff.org/mental-health/press-release/u-s-has-the-highest-rate-of-gun-deaths-for-children-and-teens-among-peer-countries/

Last, J. M. E. (2001). *A dictionary of epidemiology* (4th ed.). Oxford University Press.

Lee, L., Upadhya, K. K., Matson, P. A., Adger, H., & Trent, M. E. (2016). The status of adolescent medicine: Building a global adolescent workforce. *International Journal of Adolescent Medicine and Health, 28*(3), 233–243. https://doi.org/10.1515/ijamh-2016-5003

Lemkau, P. V. (1949). *Mental hygiene in public health* (1st ed.). Pranava Books.

Marmot, M. & Wilkinson, R.G., Editors. (1999). Social determinants of health. .

Murthy, V. H. (2021). *Protecting youth mental health: The U.S. Surgeon General's Advisory*. U.S. Department of Health and Human Services. Retrieved February 29. 2024, from https://www.hhs.gov/sites/default/files/surgeon-general-youth-mental-health-advisory.pdf

National Research Council and Institute of Medicine. (2009). *Preventing mental, emotional, and behavioral disorders among young people: Progress and possibilities* (p. 13) (Committee on the Prevention of Mental Disorders and Substance Abuse Among Children, Youth, and Young Adults: Research Advances and Promising Interventions. M. E. O'Connell, T. Boat, & K. E. Warner, Eds.). Board on Children, Youth, and Families, Division of Behavioral and Social Sciences and Education. The National Academies Press.

New York State Education Department. (2024). *Oversight of mental health education in schools*. Office of the New York State Comptroller. Retrieved May 16, 2024, from https://www.osc.ny.gov/state-agencies/audits/2022/04/11/oversight-mental-health-education-schools

Osmick, M. J., & Wilson, M. (2020). Social determinants of health—Relevant history, a call to action, an organization's transformational story, and what can employers do? *American Journal of Health Promotion, 34*(2), 219–224. https://doi.org/10.1177/0890117119896122d

Racine, N., McArthur, B. A., Cooke, J. E., Eirich, R., Zhu, J., & Madigan, S. (2021). Global prevalence of depressive and anxiety symptoms in children and adolescents during COVID-19: A meta-analysis. *JAMA Pediatrics, 175*(11), 1142–1150. https://doi.org/10.1001/jamapediatrics.2021.2482

Richards, M. C., Benson, N. M., Kozloff, N., & Franklin, M. S. (2023). Remodeling broken systems: Addressing the national emergency in child and adolescent mental health. *Psychiatric Services*. Published online 15 September. doi:https://doi.org/10.1176/appi.ps.20220283.

Schumacher, H. C. (1948). The integration of mental hygiene concepts and practices in a public health program. *Canadian Journal of Public Health, 39*(9), 351–357. https://europepmc.org/article/MED/18891228

Shultz, J. M., Sullivan, L. M., & Galea, S. (2021). *Public health: An introduction to the science and practice of population health* (1st ed., p. 59). Springer. https://www.springerpub.com/public-health-9780826177537.html#productdetails

Texas Education Agency. (n.d.). *School counseling—FAQs*. Accessed May 13, 2024, from https://tea.texas.gov/academics/learning-support-and-programs/school-guidance-and-counseling/school-counseling-faqs

The Lancet. (2016). Our future: a Lancet commission on adolescent health and wellbeing. Retrieved February 24, 2024, from https://www.thelancet.com/commissions/adolescent-health-and-wellbeing

Uhlhaas, P. J., McGorry, P. D., & Wood, S. J. (2021). Toward a paradigm for youth mental health. *JAMA Psychiatry, 78*(5), 473–474. https://jamanetwork.com/journals/jamapsychiatry/article-abstract/2774109

Uhlhaas, P. J., Davey, C. G., Mehta, U. M., et al. (2023). Towards a youth mental health paradigm: A perspective and roadmap. *Molecular Psychiatry, 28*, 3171–3181. https://doi.org/10.1038/s41380-023-02202-z

UNICEF. (2021). *The state of the world's children 2021: On my mind: promoting, protecting and caring for children's mental health.* Retrieved March 19, 2024, from https://www.unicef.org/reports/state-worlds-children-2021

UNICEF. (2023). *Investing in a safe, healthy and productive transition from childhood to adulthood is critical.* Retrieved March 19, 2024 from, https://data.unicef.org/topic/adolescents/overview/

Ventura, D. (2023, May 21). *Approximately how many parts are in a car on average?* Motor Biscuit. Retrieved May 13, 2024, from https://www.motorbiscuit.com/approximately-many-parts-car-average/

Wahlbeck, K. (2015). Public mental health: The time is ripe for translation of evidence into practice. *World Psychiatry, 14*(1), 36–42. https://doi.org/10.1002/wps.20178

Wilkinson, R., & Marmot, M. (Eds.). (1998). *Social determinants of health—The solid facts.* World Health Organization.

Williams, C. S., & Westermeyer, J. (1985). Public health aspects of mental health: The last 75 years of the American Journal of Public Health. *American Journal of Public Health, 75*(7), 722–726. https://doi.org/10.2105/ajph.75.7.722

Winslow, C. E. A. (1920). The untilled fields of public health. *Science (New York, N.Y.), 51*(1306), 23–33. https://doi.org/10.1126/science.51.1306.23

World Health Organization. (1948). *Constitution of the World Health Organization as adopted by the international health conference.* New York, 19–22 June 1946; signed on 22 July 1946 by the representatives of 61 States. Official Records of the World Health Organization (no. 2, p. 100) and entered into force on 7 April 1948. https://www.who.int/about/accountability/governance/constitution

World Health Organization. (1977). *Health needs of adolescents.* Report of a WHO Expert Committee. Technical Report Series. https://iris.who.int/handle/10665/41252

World Health Organization. (1997). *Public mental health: guidelines for the elaboration and management of national mental health programmes* (WHO/MNH/MND/96.19). https://iris.who.int/bitstream/handle/10665/63293/WHO_MNH_MND_96.19.pdf?sequence=1&isAllowed=y

World Health Organization. (2010). *A conceptual framework for action on the social determinants of health.* Retrieved April 10, 2024, from https://www.who.int/publications/i/item/9789241500852

World Health Organization. (2014). *Health for the world's adolescents: a second chance in the second decade report.* World Health Organization. Retrieved April 10, 2024, from https://www.who.int/publications/i/item/WHO-FWC-MCA-14.05

World Health Organization. (2017). *Global accelerated action for the health of adolescents (AA-HA!): Guidance to support country implementation.* Licence: CC BY-NC-SA 3.0 IGO. Retrieved April 22 2024, from https://iris.who.int/bitstream/handle/10665/255415/9789241512343-eng.pdf?sequence=1

World Health Organization. (2020). *Guidelines on mental health promotive and preventive interventions for adolescents: Helping adolescents thrive.* Introduction Available from: https://www.ncbi.nlm.nih.gov/books/NBK565368/

World Health Organization. (2021). *Fact sheet.* Mental Health of Adolescents. Retrieved, March 3, 2023, from https://www.who.int/news-room/fact-sheets/detail/adolescent-mental-health

World Health Organization. (2024). *Social determinants of health.* Retrieved March 31, 2024, from https://www.who.int/health-topics/social-determinants-of-health#tab=tab_1

World Resources Institute. (2024). *What is systems change? 6 questions answered.* Retrieve January 22, 2024, from https://www.wri.org/insights/systems-change-how-to-top-6-questions-answered

Part II
How to Make a Systems Change in Adolescent Mental Health

Chapter 5
Strategies for Implementing a Public Health Model for Adolescent Mental Health

Arthur Maerlender, Patricia Gail Bray, and Robert K. Wimpelberg

5.1 Introduction

Changing systems of care is a complex task of social engineering (or changing any "system" for that matter). Fifty years ago, leading thinkers in social design thinking felt it was an impossible task. "The search for scientific bases for confronting problems of social policy is bound to the nature of these problems. They are 'wicked' problems, whereas science has developed with 'tame' problems" (Rittel & Webber, 1973, p. 155).

However, the advent of implementation science has approached this dilemma and helped to identify strategies that address the research-to-practice gap by implementing evidence-based practices at the level of communities and regions.

Simply put, until relatively recently, the progress that has been made developing effective treatments has not been reaching communities. To address this conundrum, implementation science is providing insights into understanding heretofore unstudied elements of the process of change. Although still a young science, progress has been made for optimizing the approach to psychiatric care for youth from

A. Maerlender (✉)
Department of Psychology, Saint Anselm College, Manchester, NH, USA

Center for Brain, Biology and Behavior, University of Nebraska—Lincoln, Lincoln, NE, USA
e-mail: amaerlender@anselm.edu; amaerlender2@unl.edu

P. G. Bray
Department of Management, Policy and Community Health, UTHealth Houston School of Public Health, The University of Texas Health Science Center (UTHealth) at Houston, Houston, TX, USA
e-mail: Patricia.G.Bray@uth.tmc.edu

R. K. Wimpelberg
All Kids Alliance, College of Education, University of Houston, Houston, TX, USA
e-mail: rwimpelberg@uh.edu

P. G. Bray, A. Maerlender (eds.), *Adolescent Public Mental Health*,
https://doi.org/10.1007/978-3-031-68294-0_5

observational to experimental studies and clinical trials; identifying effective determinants; developing better targets, mechanisms of action, and outcomes; and agreeing on standardized measurements (Williams & Beidas, 2019).

This approach has led to investigations of system-elements such as attitudes and beliefs of recipients and stakeholders, organizational structure and affiliation, stages of change, skill levels and training, motivations, characteristics of implementation behaviors including frequency and sequencing of behavior, and the types of reinforcers that maintain behaviors, leadership, and resources. In short, implementation science analyzes how to direct, manage, and evaluate change at a defined population level.

This approach to thinking about systems change has led to the development and testing of different theories, approaches, and tools to facilitate better outcomes and refute Rittel and Webber's pessimistic 1973 prediction.

As articulated in this volume, the question has been how to change the trajectory of the youth mental health crisis. Consistent with WHO guidance, the goal has been to articulate a means for adapting the strengths of three systems into an efficient and effective service delivery model. These three systems are education, public health, and adolescent mental health.

5.2 Systems Change

According to Rutter et al. (2017), "A complex systems model of public health conceptualises poor health and health inequalities as outcomes of a multitude of interdependent elements within a connected whole."

A well-functioning system creates conditions for improved population health with embedded measurement to assess outcomes and the connectedness of the components. Further, aligning components or sectors in committed collaboration and evidence-driven activity and learning are key components of effective systems change (Craike et al., 2023).

According to Diez Roux (2011), complex systems are defined by several properties, including emergence, feedback, and adaptation. Emergence describes the properties of a complex system that cannot be directly predicted from the elements within it and are more than just the sum of its parts. For example, poor adolescent mental health (mental ill-health) is an emergent property of lack of prevention, social determinants of health, and family stress (to name a few elements). The effect of a single change can reinforce or create other changes in a "feedback" effect. Here an example might be the incorporation of social emotional learning improves a student's relationship with their parents that in turn leads to more supportive behavior at home that lowers stress. Adaptation refers to individual and organizational adjustments in behavior in response to the interventions.

Evaluation is a critical component of systems change. However, evaluation of research impact often assumes a linear progression from inputs to societal outcomes without linkage to higher level theory, nor does it make explicit the links between the research process and its application and contribution to societal outcomes (Craike et al., 2023).

The concept of evidence-based medicine, developing since the 1980s, has become a driving force in medicine (Mills et al., 2022) (see also Bonell et al., 2012; Cohn et al., 2013; Rhodes & Lancaster, 2019). This approach presupposes that interventions can be relatively standardizable even though they are "complicated." The randomized clinical trial (RCT) has become the standard of evidence and sharply distinguishes between intervention research and implementation science. However, a RCT approach has not been without its critics with a primary concern being the conflict between scalability of complex programs and what some researchers label "context sensitivity" or the ability to adjust models in real time to the specific local demands presented (Mills et al., 2022).

These researchers argue that successful programs should find a middle path by developing "complex, adaptive interventions that are standardized in terms of function and thus can be tested in trials despite variation in what is delivered" (Mills et al., 2022, p. 116). Achieving such a middle ground requires addressing a broader array of factors that pertain to interventions, implementation strategies, and delivery settings. These factors shape intervention effectiveness. Key findings point to robust development of implementation strategies as well as intervention activities. The implementation teams have responsibility for managing needed context-specific adaptations.

5.3 Implementation Science

Implementation science is a multidisciplinary field that focuses on understanding the processes, strategies, and factors involved in the successful integration of evidence-based practices, interventions, and policies into real-world settings. The goal of implementation science is to bridge the gap between research and practice by identifying the most effective methods for translating scientific knowledge into routine and sustainable practices in various contexts, such as healthcare, education, and public health (Bauer & Kirchner, 2020).

Mills et al. (2022) demonstrated that implementation strategies were central to complex interventions because they shape the specific forms that complex interventions take on. This ensures that adaptations remain congruent with intervention aims. One solution was to accurately characterize implementation strategies as guidelines for other projects, rather than empirical analyses and descriptions of implementation. In this way, the importance of implementation is maintained by scaling up across environments. To address the effect of tension between scalability and context sensitivity on outcomes, the concept of collective impact (CI) has emerged to facilitate effective cross-sector coordination as an antidote to the outcomes of isolated interventions of individual organizations and their constituents.

By studying the effects of specific determinants on the outcomes of evidence-based practices in child psychology and psychiatry, researchers have been able to specify important dimensions and functions within programs. For instance, at the clinical level, clinician knowledge, attitudes, and self-efficacy are important variables to attend to (Williams & Beidas, 2019). At the general organizational level, organizational culture and climate were identified (Williams & Beidas, 2019). In a more detailed review of contextual determinants, the most frequently used were organizational support, financial resources, social relations and support, and leadership which were identified as most important (Nilsen & Bernhardsson, 2019). By quantifying the effects of these determinants on outcomes, the factors that were previously suspected but not operationalized are now critical elements of processes that lead to quantifiably better outcomes.

5.4 Collective Impact

Collective impact developed out of the understanding that sustained social change is more likely to result from effective cross-sector coordination rather than from the isolated interventions of individual organizations and thus providing better context sensitivity. In their influential *Stanford Social Innovation Review* article "Collective Impact," John Kania and Mark Kramer (2011) advocated for collective impact as an effective means of working on complex social issues where no single entity has the authority or resources to bring about the necessary change. The authors note that with collective impact, the partners agree to organize their work around a common agenda, along with four other necessary conditions. Individually the partners continue to do their own work, and although they may disagree on the means toward a given set of ends, the commitment to align their work around a shared goal is a distinguishing mark of collective impact as compared to collaboration generally.

Collective impact standardizes the specific processes, guidelines, and activities for complex interventions and thus ensures that adaptations remain congruent with intervention aims. By defining a consistent process, the importance of implementation is maintained in scaling up across environments, even though specific or local outcome measures may differ.

In short, collective impact is the commitment of a group of actors from different sectors to a common agenda for solving a specific social problem, using a structured form of collaboration. In 2021, the Collective Impact Forum changed the definition of collective impact to "Collective Impact is a network of community members, organizations, and institutions who advance equity by learning together, aligning, and integrating their actions to achieve population and systems-level change" (Kania et al., 2022; Collective Impact Forum, 2022). Thus, collective impact offers a dynamic response to complex problems that meshes a particular kind of infrastructure with action processes, ever renewable and ever oriented toward the goals of sustainability, trust, and positive change at scale, as illustrated in Fig. 5.1.

In practice, all of the participants in a collective impact model have a shared vision for change, one that includes a common understanding of the problem and a

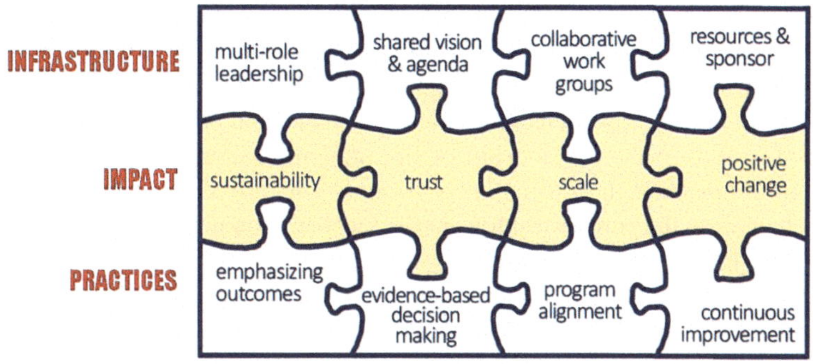

Fig. 5.1 Collective impact: relationship of infrastructure, process and outcomes. (Source. By permission from All Kids Alliance, The University of Houston, College of Education, (2019) and The Menninger Clinic)

joint approach to solving it through agreed upon action (Kania & Kramer, 2011). While sharing a common agenda is necessary, it alone is not sufficient. A second condition of collective impact is having a shared system for measuring and reporting the performance outcomes that the participants want to produce. A third condition is that, while the participants take actions that are in their areas of expertise, they do not operate in isolation; participants coordinate with and support each other. A common agenda, shared measurement system, and mutually reinforcing activities build on a foundation of trust, which requires a fourth condition—constant communication. Finally, because each participating organization typically has only enough time and resources to pursue its own purposes, a separate and fully staffed independent organization (or "backbone") is a necessary fifth condition for successful outcomes (Kania & Kramer, 2011). Box 5.1 contains a summary of the collective impact characteristics.

Box 5.1: Collective Impact Characteristics

1. All participants have a common agenda for change including a shared understanding of the problem and a joint approach to solving it through agreed upon actions
2. Collecting data and measuring results consistently across all the participants and ensures a shared measurement system for alignment and accountability
3. A plan of action that outlines and coordinates mutually reinforcing activities for each participant
4. Open and continuous communication is needed across the many players to build trust, assure mutual objectives, and create common motivation
5. A backbone organization with staff and specific set of skills to serve the entire initiative and coordinate participating organizations and agencies

Source: Kania and Kramer (2011)

Evidence for the effects of the collective impact approach comes from a study by the Collective Impact Forum of 25 CI initiatives (Spark Policy Institute and ORS Impact, 2018). The research team evaluated the extent and conditions under which the collective impact approach contributes to systems and population changes. The analysis focused on the relationship of the implementation of the *five collective impact conditions* and the *Principles of Practice* on early changes to the environments, changes to the core institutions in the local environments (systems changes), and changes in the target populations.

In general, their study identified important relationships between system level changes, population-level changes, and the core components and Principles of CI. While population-level changes could not be completely explained by CI, they were a significant contributor in 20 of 25 cases. Population changes generally stemmed from changes in services and improved practices and policies. The five sites that had demonstrated no population change had been in operation for the least amount of time. This likely had impacted their weaker implementation of the collective impact conditions and may have led to significantly fewer early changes related to partnerships. There were also significantly fewer policy changes, practice improvements, and systems change (Spark Policy Institute and ORS Impact, 2018).

One of the authors of this chapter (RW) helped implement a variation of a collective impact approach to specifically address inequities in education. The program "StriveTogether: Every Child. Cradle to Career" was developed in Cincinnati, Ohio, for communities interested in a systems approach to improving public education, namely, by using collective impact, along with two other implementation conceptual tools—theory of change (ToC) and a logic model (StriveTogether, 2024)—both of which will be discussed in the following sections.

5.5 Theory of Change

One of the earliest models of theory of change is Lewin's (1947) three step model of unfreeze, change, refreeze, which supported the idea of the need for change in order to gain improvement to existing systems (Burnes, 2020). Modern theory of change models expand this to include a statement of intentions that an organization can create to express how it wants to convert resources and processes into desired outcomes. It helps illustrate activities that lead to goals; it defines the who, where, what, and how of an intervention designed to achieve certain goals (Brest, 2009). The five characteristics of ToC are included in Box 5.2 (Taplin et al., 2013).

Box 5.2: Characteristics of Theories of Change

1. The nature and sources of the problem or opportunity that require a change
2. The vision of the desired results or impact
3. The activities or strategies that will be implemented to address the problem or opportunity
4. The outcomes or changes that are expected to occur as a result of the activities or strategies
5. The assumptions or beliefs that underlie the theory of change

Source: Taplin et al. (2013)

A ToC is project-specific and related to evaluation. It makes the underlying rationale of a project explicit, which supports planning, implementation, and assessment of the project. Additionally, funding agencies often require an explicit ToC as part of a grant proposal. Reinholz and Andrews (2020) distinguish between a theory of change and a change theory. Change theories represent theoretical and empirically grounded knowledge about how change occurs that goes beyond any one project. Ideally, a ToC is informed by a change theory.

As a tool of project-specific change, a ToC recognizes that many intermediate changes in condition—or results—may be needed to reach a goal. ToC defines and diagrams those intermediate ends in causal pathways. In doing so, ToC provides the means of measuring and reporting progress in the early and middle stages of the initiative, where modifications can be made more easily (MacKinnon et al., 2006).

Additionally, a ToC articulates the vision of processes and practices that guides implementation. But large-scale prevention and intervention programs are by nature complex and often involve multiple constituencies. These often require different implementation and delivery processes that lead to different local outcomes, even if the larger program outcomes are consistent. Logic models provide specificity to the ToC.

A theory of change is a critical tool to help programs illustrate their activities and goals and to make explicit the intention of the proposed initiative together with the expected changes. Developing such a theory is a critical step in creating systems change (Craike et al., 2023). For program evaluators, understanding a program's intended progression from intervention (challenge) to outcomes (impacts) drives evaluation questions and evaluation plan development (Sharp, 2021). An example of how ToC moves from challenge to impact is illustrated in Fig. 5.2.

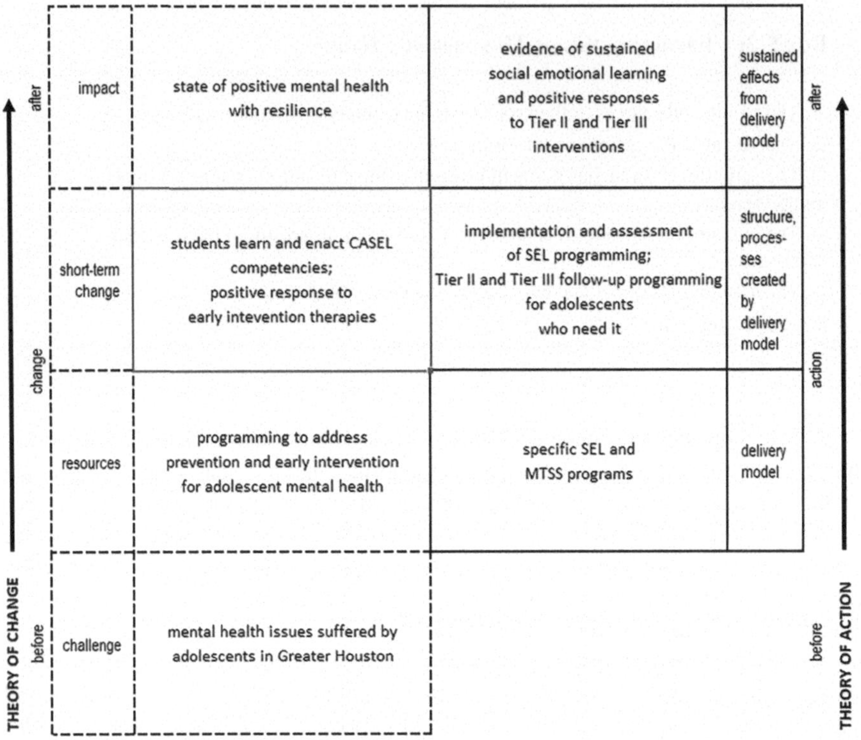

Fig. 5.2 Example: theories of change from challenge to impact. (Source. By permission from All Kids Alliance, The University of Houston, College of Education, (2019) and The Menninger Clinic)

5.6 Logic Models

Although similar to a ToC, a logic model is based on a logical sequence of steps (Baxter et al., 2018, 2020; Craig et al., 2008). On the other hand, as its name implies, a theory of change is theory-driven. The mechanisms responsible for how the various components interact with each other can develop from real-world examples, academic literature, or even program leaders' hypotheses. Because of this difference, a logic model is usually constructed after the program is developed, as a way of describing the program and its intended outcomes, while a theory of change is most useful when considered before program development as a way to determine the best intervention(s) for the desired outcome(s). This is not always the case in practice but nonetheless reflects the individual strengths of both the ToC and logic models (Sharp, 2021).

The intention of using logic models is to build understanding and clarity about the program, identify resources needed, specify the sequencing of activities that should be implemented, and thus serve as a basis for program evaluation. Logic models articulate a process for measuring outcomes. They should describe the chain of causes and effects leading to an outcome of interest (e.g., creating processes for prevention and early intervention for adolescent mental illness). Logic models are helpful for program evaluation by providing a picture of how the program is intended to work (Centers for Disease Control, n.d.).

However, the logic model is more than a graphical depiction: Included are the theories, scientific evidence, assumptions, and beliefs that support the logic model and the various processes behind it. Logic *modeling* is a technique that "encourages iterative development of an idea, program or project" (Knowlton & Phillips, 2012).

One logic modeling approach is called intervention mapping, a protocol for developing theory-based and evidence-based health promotion programs (Bartholomew et al., 1998). Intervention mapping, first developed in 1998, was a reaction to a lack of comprehensive frameworks for health promotion program development and describes the process of health promotion program planning in six steps (Bartholomew et al., 1998). The six steps are described below and listed in Box 5.3:

1. A needs assessment based cost-benefit analyses.
2. A definition of performance and change objectives based upon scientific analyses of health problems and problem causing factors.
3. A selection of theory-based intervention methods and practical applications to change (determinants of) health-related behavior.
4. A description of program components, design, and production.
5. The anticipated timing of program adoption, implementation, and sustainability.
6. The anticipated process and effectiveness and sustainability of the program in an evaluation plan.

Box 5.3: Characteristics of Logic Models

1. Inputs (resources)
2. Activities (strategies, events)
3. Outputs (products of activities)
4. Short-term outcomes (immediate effects: weeks-months)
5. Intermediate-term outcomes (intended effects over the midterm: months-years)
6. Long-term outcomes (long-term intended effects: years-decades)

Source: Bartholomew et al. (1998)

5.7 Distinctions Between Logic Models and Theory of Change

Although the terms "logic model" and "theory of change" are often used interchangeably, there are some key differences that affect how they are developed and used.

Sharp (2021) makes a distinction between a logic model and theory of change: A logic model describes a logical sequence showing the intervention's intended outcomes, whereas a ToC articulates the causality and why each intervention component is expected to result in the intended outcomes. However, contextual factors and assumptions can be included in a logic model. Thus, a logic model is descriptive while a theory of change is explanatory. Furthermore, theory of change mechanisms are accessible to empirical analysis providing a basis for demonstrating effect. This is not a trivial matter as systems change should be based on solid evidence (Craike et al., 2023).

The progression of steps is also described differently between logic models and theories of change. Logic models tend to be linear and progress in a step-by-step manner starting with inputs to activities and to impact, moving from cause to effect. Components of a theory of change are not always linear and effects may influence later causes.

5.8 Rapid Cycle Improvement

An important tool that can assist in the management of logic models and theories of change is to implement *rapid cycle improvement*. Rapid cycle improvement (RCI) is a "quality improvement method that identifies, implements and measures changes made to improve a process or a system" (The Office of the National Coordinator for Health Information Technology, 2019). RCI implies that changes are made and tested over periods of 3 months or less, rather than the standard 6–12 months. RCI is the continuous process of defining, monitoring, and measuring program improvement. Measurement is included within each level of implementation; thus, it is called "rapid cycle."

Each element of the logic model has a defined measurement tool and process. Implementing and maintaining this process is not without its drawbacks. A top-down approach to the establishment of tools and procedures can alienate staff. Therefore, those required to use measurement and observation tools should be involved in the decision-making. Further, the standards used for measurement can be difficult to define. A lowest common denominator of expectation may be the only place to start and still get consensus. RCI can be time-consuming, and frontline staff need the time to collect and report the respective data points. Additionally, monthly meetings can be burdensome to overworked and underpaid staff. Further, measurement assumes comparison, and staff may be defensive about being judged on things they have little control over. Leadership must, therefore, create an environment of collaboration and cooperation that supports staff in these efforts, since quality improvement processes are dependent upon them (Agency for Healthcare Research and Quality, 2020a).

One approach to implementing rapid cycle improvement that was implemented in 1995 is called the Consumer Assessment of Healthcare Providers and Systems (CAHPS). Box 5.4 provides an exemplar of rapid cycle improvement. CAHPS is a registered trademark of the Agency for Healthcare Research and Quality (AHRQ), which provides general guidance for implementing quality improvement procedures (Agency for Healthcare Research and Quality, 2020a, c).

Box 5.4: Rapid Cycle Exemplar

The CAHPS survey is used as the gold standard for program effectiveness and ongoing RCI. AHRQ provides three tips for facilitating the quality improvement process, which include the following:

1. A priority is placed on encouraging communication, engagement, and participation for all of the stakeholders affected by the QI [quality improvement] process. This includes learning what is most important to the people who make up the microsystem and looking for ways to help take responsibility and ownership of the changes.
2. Implementation of improvements should start with small-scale demonstrations, which are easier to manage than large-scale changes. Small-scale demonstrations or small tests of change also allow refinement of new processes and demonstration of their impact on existing practices and outcomes and build increased support by all stakeholders.
3. Quality improvement is an iterative process and this message may need frequent repetition. It is not unusual to make frequent corrections along the way as experience with each step helps to identify other actions to improve strategy.

Source: Agency for Healthcare Research and Quality (2020a, c)

The specific tools should be validated and demonstrate adequate reliability so that cross-program comparisons can be made. Validation can be in the form of a group of subject matter experts agreeing on items and then testing the items in a sample to assure its performance. This is consistent with the Plan-Action-Study-Do model, which is part of RCI (Agency for Healthcare Research and Quality, 2020b). The team responsible for implementation should have access to measurement and subject matter experts to support their efforts. An example of the relationship between logic models and RCI is illustrated in Fig. 5.3.

LOGIC MODEL: ***Rapid Cycle Continuous Improvement***			**measuring success**		
EFFORTS		>	EFFECTS		
Processes		>	Short-Term ⟶	**Outcomes**	⟶ Long-Term
What are the main **Activities** you are employing?	What will be the **Outputs** of your activities?	>	What will **Learning** look like?	What **Behavior Change** will take place?	What **Impact** will that learning and behavior change have?
informal assessment of adequacy of preparation and training for interventions	*student attendance during Tier I, Tier II, and/or Tier III activities* *informal gauge of student engagement during activities* *informal assessment of quality of program delivery: fidelity to training; clarity of guidance*	> > > > >	*survey of students' knowledge of terms and their meaning* *observations of students' social emotional language during Tier I, Tier II, and Tier III activities*	*informal observations of students' behavior* *monitoring of students' grades and discipline referrals*	*cumulative, multi-year review of data gathered around learning and behavior change*

Fig. 5.3 (Example) Logic model and rapid cycle continuous improvement: measuring success—activities, outputs, learning, behavior change, and impact. (By permission from All Kids Alliance, The University of Houston, College of Education, (2000) and The Menninger Clinic)

5.9 Conclusion

Implementation science has provided the clinical world valuable theories, lessons, and determinants for increasing the effectiveness and sustainability of large-scale interventions. By taking a public health approach to mental illness prevention, the "marriage" of community mental health to community schools to utilize evidence-based practices at a population level is now a realistic possibility. When implemented, these heuristic models hold significant promise for improving mental health outcomes, particularly for adolescents.

As the case study in the next chapter demonstrates, the collective impact approach utilizing theory of change, logic models, and rapid cycle improvement appears to be a successful implementation of a multisectoral and multi-stakeholder approach to prevention and care of adolescent well-being and mental health challenges.

Competing Interests

1. *The BridgeUp at Menninger study was generously funded by the David and Helen Gurley Brown Trust, BridgeUp: Mental Health at The Menninger Clinic.*

2. Patricia Gail Bray *has received consultant fees from* The Menninger Clinic, located in Houston, Texas.
3. Robert Wimpelberg *has received consultant fees from* The Menninger Clinic, located in Houston, Texas.

References

Agency for Healthcare Research and Quality. (2020a, January). *Section 4: Ways to approach the quality improvement process*. https://www.ahrq.gov/cahps/quality-improvement/improvement-guide/4-approach-qi-process/index.html#4b

Agency for Healthcare Research and Quality. (2020b, September). *Plan-Do-Study-Act (PDSA) directions and examples*. Retrieved January 6, 2024, from https://www.ahrq.gov/health-literacy/improve/precautions/tool2b.html

Agency for Healthcare Research and Quality. (2020c). *CAHPS: Surveys and tools to advance patient-centered care*. Retrieved June 11, 2024, from https://www.ahrq.gov/cahps/index.html

Bartholomew, L. K., Parcel, G. S., & Kok, G. (1998). Intervention mapping: A process for developing theory and evidence-based health education programs. *Health Education & Behavior, 25*(5), 545–563. https://doi.org/10.1177/109019819802500502

Bauer, M. S., & Kirchner, J. (2020). Implementation science: What is it and why should I care? *Psychiatry Research, 283*, 112376. https://doi.org/10.1016/j.psychres.2019.04.025

Baxter, R., O'Hara, J., Murray, J., Sheard, L., Cracknell, A., Foy, R., Wright, J., & Lawton, R. (2018). Partners at care transitions: Exploring healthcare professionals' perspectives of excellence at care transitions for older people. *BMJ Open, 8*(9), e022468. https://doi.org/10.1136/bmjopen-2018-022468

Baxter, R., Murray, J., O'Hara, J., Hewitt, C., Richardson, G., Cockayne, S., Sheard, L., Mills, T., & Lawton, R. (2020). Improving patient experience and safety at transitions of care through the your care needs you (YCNY) intervention: A study protocol for a cluster randomised controlled feasibility trial. *Pilot and Feasibility Studies, 6*(1). https://doi.org/10.1186/s40814-020-00655-5

Bonell, C., Fletcher, A., Morton, M., Lorenc, T., & Moore, L. (2012). Realist randomised controlled trials: A new approach to evaluating complex public health interventions. *Social Science & Medicine, 75*(12), 2299–2306. https://doi.org/10.1016/j.socscimed.2012.08.032

Brest, P. (2009, Spring). The power of theories of change. *Stanford Social Innovation Review*. https://ssir.org/articles/entry/the_power_of_theories_of_change

Burnes, B. (2020). The origins of Lewin's three-step model of change. *The Journal of Applied Behavioral Science, 56*(1), 32–59. https://doi.org/10.1177/0021886319892685

Centers for Disease Control. (n.d.). *Identifying the components of a logic model*. https://www.cdc.gov/std/Program/pupestd/Components%20of%20a%20Logic%20Model.pdf

Cohn, S., Clinch, M., Bunn, C., & Stronge, P. (2013). Entangled complexity: Why complex interventions are just not complicated enough. *Journal of Health Services Research & Policy, 18*(1), 40–43. https://doi.org/10.1258/jhsrp.2012.012036

Collective Impact Forum. (2022, April 14). *What is collective impact*. Retrieved November 13, 2023, from https://collectiveimpactforum.org/what-is-collective-impact/

Craig, P., Dieppe, P., MacIntyre, S., Michie, S., Nazareth, I., & Petticrew, M. (2008). Developing and evaluating complex interventions: The new Medical Research Council guidance. *The BMJ, a1655*. https://doi.org/10.1136/bmj.a1655

Craike, M., Klepac, B., Mowle, A., & Riley, T. (2023). Theory of systems change: An initial, middle-range theory of public health research impact. *Research Evaluation, 32*(3), 603–621. https://doi.org/10.1093/reseval/rvad030

Diez Roux, A. V. (2011). Complex systems thinking and current impasses in health disparities research. *American Journal of Public Health, 101*, 1627–1634.

Kania, J., & Kramer, M. (2011, Winter). Collective impact. *Stanford Social Innovation Review*. https://ssir.org/articles/entry/collective_impact

Kania, J., Williams, J., Schmitz, P., Brady, S., Kramer, M., & Juster, J. S. (2022, Winter). Centering equity in collective impact. *Stanford Social Innovation Review*. Retrieved February 7, 2024, from https://ssir.org/articles/entry/centering_equity_in_collective_impact

Knowlton, L. W., & Phillips, C. C. (2012). Chapter 1. Introducing logic models. In *The logic model guidebook: Better strategies for great results*. Sage Publications. Retrieved April 2, 2024, from https://www.sagepub.com/sites/default/files/upm-binaries/50363_ch_1.pdf

Lewin, K. (1947). Frontiers in group dynamics: Concept, method and reality in social science; social equilibria and social change. *Human Relations, 1*(1), 5–41.

MacKinnon, A., Amott, N., & McGarvey, C. (2006). Mapping change: Using a theory of change to guide planning and evaluation. *Candid Learning for Funders*. https://learningforfunders.candid.org/wp-content/uploads/sites/2/2018/12/theory_change.pdf

Mills, T., Shannon, R., O'Hara, J., Lawton, R., & Sheard, L. (2022). Development of a 'real-world' logic model through testing the feasibility of a complex healthcare intervention: The challenge of reconciling scalability and context-sensitivity. *Evaluation, 28*(1), 113–131. https://doi.org/10.1177/13563890211068869

Nilsen, P., & Bernhardsson, S. (2019). Context matters in implementation science: A scoping review of determinant frameworks that describe contextual determinants for implementation outcomes. *BMC Health Services Research, 19*, 189. https://doi.org/10.1186/s12913-019-4015-3

Reinholz, D. L., & Andrews, T. C. (2020). Change theory and theory of change: what's the difference anyway? *International Journal of STEM Education, 7*(1). https://doi.org/10.1186/s40594-020-0202-3

Rhodes, T., & Lancaster, K. (2019). Evidence-making interventions in health: A conceptual framing. *Social Science & Medicine, 238*, 112488. https://doi.org/10.1016/j.socscimed.2019.112488

Rittel, H. W. J., & Webber, M. M. (1973). Dilemmas in a general theory of planning. *Policy Sciences, 4*(2), 155–169.

Rutter, H., Savona, N., Glonti, K., Bibby, J., Cummins, S., Finegood, D. T., Greaves, F., Harper, L., Hawe, P., Moore, L., Petticrew, M., Rehfuess, E., Shiell, A., Thomas, J., & White, M. (2017). The need for a complex systems model of evidence for public health. *Lancet, 390*(10112), 2602–2604. https://doi.org/10.1016/S0140-6736(17)31267-9

Sharp. (2021, March 15). *Logic models vs theories of change*. Center for Research Evaluation. https://cere.olemiss.edu/logic-models-vs-theories-of-change/.

Spark Policy Institute and ORS Impact. (2018). *When collective impact has an impact: A cross-site study of 25 collective impact initiatives*. Retrieved April 2, 2024, from https://collectiveimpactforum.org/wp-content/uploads/2021/12/CI-Study-Report.pdf.

StriveTogether. (2024). *Strive together: Every child. cradle to career.* Retrieved February 7, 2024, from https://www.strivetogether.org/

Taplin, D. H., Clark, H., Collins, E., & Colb, D. C. (2013, April). *Theory of change: A series of papers to support development of theories of change based on practice in the field*. ActKnowledge. https://www.theoryofchange.org/wp-content/uploads/toco_library/pdf/ToC-Tech-Papers.pdf

The Office of the National Coordinator for Health Information Technology. (2019, April 19). *How do I use a rapid-cycle improvement strategy?* HealthIT.gov. https://www.healthit.gov/faq/how-do-i-use-rapid-cycle-improvement-strategy

Williams, N. J., & Beidas, R. S. (2019). Annual research review: The state of implementation science in child psychology and psychiatry: A review and suggestions to advance the field. *Journal of Child Psychology and Psychiatry, 60*(4), 430–450. https://doi.org/10.1111/jcpp.12960

Chapter 6
BridgeUp Case Study: The BridgeUp Model Implementation

Patricia Gail Bray, Arthur Maerlender, and Robert K. Wimpelberg

6.1 Introduction Background

This chapter features the design, development, implementation, and evaluation of the David and Helen Gurley Brown BridgeUp: Mental Health Center, which is the basis for the BridgeUp Center (BridgeUp) at The Menninger Clinic (Menninger) Case Study. The Menninger Clinic, located in Houston, Texas, is a nationally ranked leader in psychiatry. BridgeUp was made possible with a generous gift from the David and Helen Gurley Brown Trust, now the Helen Gurley Brown Foundation (HGB), in New York.

Supplementary Information The online version contains supplementary material available at https://doi.org/10.1007/978-3-031-68294-0_6.

P. G. Bray (✉)
Department of Management, Policy and Community Health, UTHealth Houston School of Public Health, The University of Texas Health Science Center (UTHealth) at Houston, Houston, TX, USA
e-mail: Patricia.G.Bray@uth.tmc.edu

A. Maerlender
Department of Psychology, Saint Anselm College, Manchester, NH, USA

Center for Brain, Biology and Behavior, University of Nebraska—Lincoln, Lincoln, NE, USA
e-mail: amaerlender@anselm.edu

R. K. Wimpelberg
All Kids Alliance, College of Education, University of Houston, Houston, TX, USA
e-mail: rwimpelberg@uh.edu

P. G. Bray, A. Maerlender (eds.), *Adolescent Public Mental Health*,
https://doi.org/10.1007/978-3-031-68294-0_6

BridgeUp was formed with a small group of experienced staff responsible for the 7-year demonstration project. The mission of BridgeUp was "to create bold, sustainable systemic improvements that bolster mental health, well-being, academic achievement and social and emotional learning in vulnerable adolescents" (BridgeUp at Menninger, 2017, p. 1). With the HGB funding, the BridgeUp leadership team sought guidance from distinguished health leaders, innovators, and educators across the community, including from the Texas Medical Center's (TMC) member institutions. This diverse group served as the BridgeUp Advisory Committee (AC) during the formative pilot years, 2015–2019. The charge from HGB for the funding was to create a "disruptive" and "transformative" mental health model and program for underserved adolescents living in the Greater Houston area.

The HGB Board, and the Menninger CEO and Board, provided program oversight, with Dr. Bray serving as liaison between the two groups in the executive director role. HGB, Menninger, and the AC agreed on the structure of the model to be implemented in schools, which included a public health approach (National Academies of Sciences, Engineering, and Medicine, et al., 2019) and a collective impact approach (Kania & Kramer, 2011), which are explained below. Certainly, for the schools located in the Houston region, few schools were interested in formalizing a public health approach for adolescent mental health, and most were not aware of collective impact. This meant that the BridgeUp model and program would be disruptive and—at the end of the project—transformative.

6.1.1 Magic Grants Funding

With the funding secured through the HGB Foundation, Dr. Bray began the search for community partners interested in developing a school mental health prevention model with generously funded community grants. A request for proposal (RFP) process was developed and disseminated through social media sites, professional networks, and academic institutions, such as the University of Texas Health Science Center's Houston School of Public Health, local medical schools, and a collaborative for school-based mental health that included 48 regional school districts and mental health providers. An orientation session was held for those who responded, and a letter of intent to participate was requested. The school principals and intended grant leads were then interviewed at which time the grant proposal structure and grant deliverables were described.

The submitted grants, called *Magic Grants*, were anonymously reviewed by a group of community and healthcare leaders and scored using a predefined rubric. After scoring, the anonymous community-based review team met to discuss scoring and to make final Magic Grants selections. An average of seven programs participated in the annual grant process. Previously awarded programs who were eligible could reapply for another year of funding. Magic Grants applications for funding were evaluated according to the BridgeUp evaluation plan featuring the BridgeUp model components, along with proposed student and school outcomes.

6.1.2 BridgeUp Model Principles

There are five principles that constitute the BridgeUp model. These principles are not meant to stand alone. These principles become an integrated whole, which is a consistent theme woven throughout not only the model structure but the implementation of the model. The BridgeUp five principles serve as the basis for the new adolescent public mental health model that was presented in an earlier chapter of this volume.

Principle 1 is the framing of the BridgeUp model intentionally with a broader social ecological (SE) model, which expands the definition of health to include more than absence of disease. As the Centers for Disease Control and Prevention (CDC, 2022) note, an SE model accounts for the "complex interplay between individual, relationship, community, and societal factors" (CDC, 2022; See also, Dahlberg & Krug, 2002).

In just the past few decades, developments related to the social ecosystem have led to fundamental shifts in the research and practice of health (including mental health) and health equity. A newer take on the SE model expands the scope to include eight ever wider circles of influence, including the individual, family, social network, neighborhood, city, state, country, and global levels (Shultz et al., 2021, p. 5).

Principle 2 builds on the SE model by using strategies regarding a public health approach, which necessarily addresses both the individual and the population levels of health. Improving adolescents will improve the entire population of adolescents. A public health approach includes the integration of the social determinants of health (Marmot & Wilkinson, 1999) and the three prevention tiers of public health, including the primary, secondary, and tertiary tiers.

Principle 3 adopts the CDC's Healthy Schools (2023) *Whole School, Whole Community and Whole Child* (WSCC) approach. The CDC's WSCC framework recognizes the connections between health, school, community, families, and the students, with the acknowledgment of the multifaceted influences that nurture the health and education of the whole child/adolescent. The WSCC approach aligns with the SE model regarding adolescent mental health and schools. A holistic view of the whole child/adolescent was integrated into the development of the BridgeUp model because there is no health without mental health.

This approach has many possible applications, and BridgeUp chose the Michigan University's Department of Education's definition of "whole child" to guide the design and implementation of the BridgeUp program (University of Michigan Department of Education, n.d.). Thus, whole child/adolescent is defined as "a unique learner comprised of interacting dimensions such as cognitive, physical, behavioral, social, and emotional. The whole child/adolescent lives within multiple and interconnected environments including home, school, and community." A holistic approach to health leads to prevention and the treatment of illness as part of the whole person and benefits the whole population.

Principle 4 supports the creation and implementation of a new model in schools that is based on a public health approach, defined in Principle 2, which means an expansion to the adolescent mental health system, that is focused primarily on disease diagnosis and treatment. An early advocate defines a public health approach as including prevention, screening, treatment, and environmental and social interventions (Stiffman et al., 2010). The National Academies of Sciences, Engineering and Medicine (2019) published a consensus study titled, *Promoting Positive Adolescent Health Behaviors and Outcomes: Thriving in the twenty-first Century*. One of their preferred frameworks is the public health prevention framework, which includes the following:

1. Primary prevention, such as teaching mental health literacy.
2. Secondary prevention, which promotes early identification of diseases or conditions, such as mental disorders.
3. Tertiary prevention, which includes treatment and management, such as with a mental illness disease.

Additionally, integrated into Principle 4 are the social determinants of health (SDOH), which address health equity by expanding health to include the application of nonmedical factors (Marmot & Wilkinson, 1999).

Principle 5 fosters what Kania and Kramer (2011) call *collective impact* (CI). This involves bringing a multisector collaboration together in a structured way to achieve systems and social change. BridgeUp's agenda included changing and improving the adolescent mental health system by integrating overlapping features of the public health, mental health, and school health systems. Due to the inherent challenges found within complex system change initiatives, the authors noted the conundrum that "large-scale social change requires broad cross-sector coordination, yet the social sector remains focused on the isolated intervention of individual organizations" (Kania & Kramer, 2011). The BridgeUp model aims to explicitly attend to this challenge.

Health equity is a common core theme embedded within each of these principles, and by using a collective impact approach, health equity is integrated within the BridgeUp model (Ackerman-Barger et al., 2020; Kania et al., 2022). The development of the BridgeUp model followed the collective impact forum's (Kania, et al., 2022; Collective Impact Forum, 2022) five strategies to center equity as included in Box 6.1.

Box 6.1: Collective Impact's Equity Strategies

- Ground the work in data and context
- Focus on systems change, programs and services
- Shift power within the collaborative
- Listen to and act with the community
- Build equity leadership and accountability

Source: Kania, et al., 2022, Collective Impact Forum, 2022

The collective impact research included the long-standing StriveTogether Network, which uses a collective impact approach to improve educational outcomes (StriveTogether, n.d.). One of the founding members of the StriveTogether National Advisory Board (RW) served on the BridgeUp leadership team, helping to establish the BridgeUp model implementation during both the Pilot Phase I (2016–2019) and the Sustainability Phase II (2019–2022). Additionally, two other BridgeUp leadership team members had prior experience working with healthcare systems in the TMC using a CI approach, along with the four other principles.

Therefore, the BridgeUp model's basic structure includes the adoption of a CI approach; integration with a public health approach, including prevention and the SDOH; and the inclusion of both population and individual levels, the WSCC framework, and the social ecological model.

6.2 Adolescent Mental Health System Change

The principles constituting the BridgeUp model were formed during the past three decades from the research in adolescent mental health, public health, and education. Building on that science, significant advances in the adolescent mental health system have occurred post-pandemic. What has changed since COVID-19 is an alignment or convergence of thought among the primary systems that intersect with the adolescent mental health system, which includes the public health and school health systems. Timing is important as to how well system change will be accepted and adapted. This convergence, along with the declarations by the surgeon general and the associated professions, discussed in earlier chapters, indicates that an adolescent mental health system change is timely.

Fortunately, the implementation of the BridgeUp model began before the pandemic, and the project was completed post-pandemic, with favorable outcomes and limited disruptions.

6.3 The BridgeUp Model Overview

Generating positive academic, social, emotional, behavioral, and mental health outcomes, the BridgeUp model serves as the basis for a possible solution to the adolescent mental health crisis and a motivation for this book.

Evidence guided early model development, including research from the Institute of Medicine (IOM); the World Health Organization; the National Academies of Sciences, Engineering and Medicine (NAS); the Centers for Disease Control and Prevention (CDC); and other public, mental, and school health research. This work was developed prior to ESSA and 4 years before COVID-19, and consequently, the landscape looked very different than it does today. There has been much more

Box 6.2: The BridgeUp Model

1. Mental health literacy: uses a social and emotional learning (SEL) platform from the Collaborative for Academic, Social and Emotional Learning (CASEL) (CASEL, n.d.-a)
2. Public health's prevention and early intervention approach: includes school-defined protocols for student screening and referrals to Tiers 2 and 3 (Center on Multi-Tiered System of Supports, n.d.)
3. Multisector collaboration: uses a collective impact approach for solving complex system challenges (Kania & Kramer, 2011).

attention and advancement to adolescent mental health, although focused more on the problems than the solutions.

The peer-reviewed and gray literature contributed to the model framework. Additionally, the team had personal communication with scholars and nonprofit leaders on the cutting edge of public health, mental health literacy and prevention, and school health integration. Included were those working in the early years of social emotional learning (SEL) (Sugai & Horner, 2009; Sugai, 2018), multitiered system of supports (MTSS), collective impact, and school mental health in the USA, including Roger Weissberg, University of Illinois, personal communication, 2015; George Sugai, University of Connecticut, personal communication, 2015; FSG, Dallas Consulting Group, personal communication, 2016; Larry Cohen, Prevention Institute, 2015; and Cynthia Briggs, President, Communities in Schools (Houston), 2015, among many others.

The development of the preventive intervention model included integrating public health knowledge of the leadership team with Menninger's expertise as a premier psychiatric health system for almost 100 years. The resulting BridgeUp model is an evidence-based, multisector, collaborative, public health approach to improving adolescent mental health in the underserved Houston areas. The model components are described as follows in Box 6.2.

6.4 The BridgeUp Model: Integration of Three Evidence-Based Frameworks

The three BridgeUp frameworks were implemented in schools during the inaugural academic year (2016–2017), with various programming approaches, depending on the culture, diversity, and size of the school. The combination of implementing mental health literacy through CASEL's SEL framework as primary prevention and providing mental health supports for secondary and tertiary prevention as part of the MTSS framework proved to work well with the multisector partnerships. Incorporating the collective impact framework together with SEL and MTSS was a

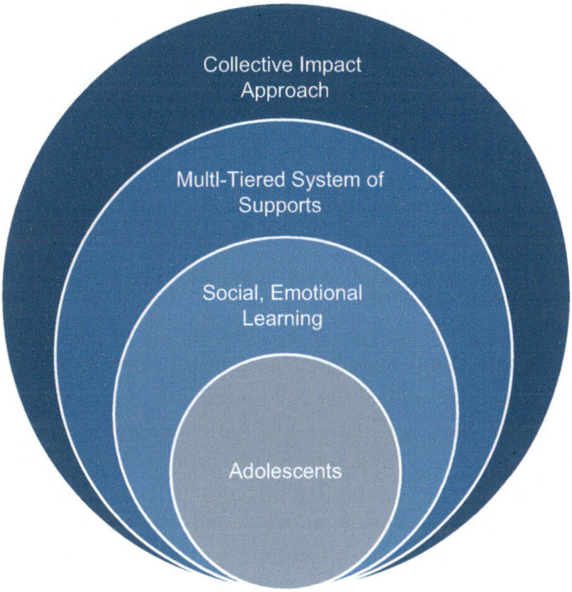

Fig. 6.1 The BridgeUp model—prevention, intervention, and multisector collaboration. (Adapted and used by Permission from The Menninger Clinic)

distinctive departure from adolescent mental health in schools in the Houston area. These three evidence-based frameworks are illustrated in Fig. 6.1.

During the preliminary research phase, the surprise was that the schools in the area that were concerned about adolescent mental health used SEL *or* MTSS, but never both. That has changed since COVID-19, as reported in the school health chapter. Although multisectoral collaboration is becoming more recognized in healthcare (Schor, 2024), especially since COVID-19, the addition of collective impact was a true innovation for the model and one of the primary reasons for BridgeUp's success. The description of each of the frameworks and how they were implemented during the Pilot Phase I is discussed in the next section.

6.4.1 BridgeUp Model's Primary Prevention Framework: Mental Health Literacy Using Social Emotional Learning

Educating adolescents about mental health literacy is based on classical public health primary prevention (National Center for Environmental Health, 2017). Mental health literacy is regarded as particularly critical for youth in their early adolescence (Nobre et al., 2021). Social and emotional learning (SEL) is one approach to addressing mental health literacy in adolescents, particularly in schools

(CASEL, n.d.-c). The universal application of SEL is a validated approach to improving mental health literacy by building mental, social, and emotional life skills and effective behavioral responses to stress and challenges that too often undermine student success (Durlak et al., 2015; Black, 2021).

After review of existing school SEL platforms, the BridgeUp leadership team chose the Collaborative for Academic, Social and Emotional Learning (CASEL) platform (CASEL, 2021). For the past two decades, CASEL has been a leader in developing the research for SEL programs defined as the acquisition of knowledge, skills, attitudes, and empathy and the ability to maintain healthy relationships and good decision-making (CASEL, n.d.-c).

CASEL was chosen as the BridgeUp SEL platform due to five primary reasons. First, this platform provided the comprehensiveness of the curricula to build social and emotional competencies and skills that correlate with the SEL definition: self-awareness, social awareness, self-management, relationship skills, and responsible decision-making. These five competencies are represented in what is called the CASEL-5 wheel, which includes the five SEL competencies and their relationship with classrooms, schools, families, caregivers, and communities (CASEL, n.d.-a). Additionally, the competencies are taken into consideration with aligned learning opportunities and authentic partnerships within the schoolwide and classroom culture, practices, and policies.

Second, CASEL has extensive research and experience working directly in the classrooms and schools. The BridgeUp model began the first pilot with after-school and in-school classes held in mostly secondary schools. Third, the CASEL framework acknowledged the importance of collaboration, which fits squarely with the model's collective impact framework. Fourth, from a public health point of view, an expanded social ecological system is vital to the success of any transformative initiative, and CASEL's approach attended to students, families, schools, and communities. They note that "the principles of SEL are present in every caring, collaborative relationship and live in the partnerships between students, schools, families, and communities throughout history" (Collaborative for Academic, Social and Emotional Learning, n.d.-b).

This leads to the fifth reason that the CASEL platform was adopted as part of the BridgeUp model: the importance of seeing the whole child and the environment in which the child lives. This was a critical concern for the model, since the original charge of the initiative was to work in underserved communities. With equity as a core value of the BridgeUp model, it was imperative to understand the implications for adolescent mental health with poverty and education and the other social determinants of health. The CASEL-5 wheel depicts concisely all of the reasons why this was a good fit with the BridgeUp model.

A primary aim for the BridgeUp model was for the grants to advance the CASEL framework for school and student success. After year 1, school-based SEL programs were required to use CASEL for the implementation of the model. Additionally, in alignment with the evolving research, further requirements stipulated that the Magic Grants recipients were required to provide the following:

Box 6.3: CASEL Endorsed SEL Program Examples
Second Step is a research-based curricula endorsed by CASEL (Second Step, 2024). Social and emotional skills learned include the following:

- Empathy
- Emotional management
- Problem-solving
- Communication
- Relationship building

The Fourth R is a research-based curricula endorsed by CASEL (The Fourth R, 2024). Program features include the following:

- Evidence-based approach
- Integration of SEL into school curriculum
- Improved other SEL skills and attitudes
- Teacher training and support
- Comprehensive approach

Training and coaching for teachers, administrators, and other school-related personnel to build SEL competence and capacity to teach and model SEL.

Educational initiatives that reinforce SEL instruction, supported by community partnerships.

Universal SEL programs and activities for all students in the target population, ideally schoolwide (target population began as an after-school program in the inaugural year and incrementally moved to include the entire school and school districts).

Further, classroom-based programming should use evidence-informed curriculum and instruction that is aligned with CASEL.

Box 6.3 includes a sampling of CASEL endorsed SEL programs for middle school that were used by selected BridgeUp programs (Second Step, 2024; The Fourth R, 2024).

6.4.2 BridgeUp Model's Secondary and Tertiary Framework: Multitiered System of Supports

The second part of the BridgeUp model includes the multitiered system of supports (MTSS) and is based on public health's prevention model, which includes the development of customized school protocols to identify and refer students who need additional mental health supports. MTSS was recommended by the U.S. Department of Education (2011) in a memo with the intention of helping at-risk students: "With a multitiered instructional framework, schools identify students at-risk for poor learning outcomes, monitor student progress, provide evidence-based interventions, and adjust the intensity and nature of those interventions depending on a student's responsiveness" (Musgrove, 2011, cited in U.S. Department of Education (2011).

Since 2011, schools using MTSS has been refined and expanded. The image in Fig. 6.2 is from the Massachusetts Department of Elementary and Secondary Education (2023), which is an exemplar of integrated adolescent mental health concepts. Included is a universal design for learning equitable access. The meaning of the three tiers hasn't changed, yet the focus on academic, behavioral, and the social emotional, speaks to the advancement of MTSS since the BridgeUp model inception in 2015.

Schools often have multiple initiatives aimed at promoting student achievement and well-being. A multitiered system of support is required to help align these programs. Additionally, behavioral and mental health needs must be identified, assessed, and addressed for students at-risk or already experiencing social, emotional, and/or behavioral difficulties.

Adopting this approach was intended to reduce the need for expensive evaluations and to focus on prevention instead. The enrollment targets are aspirational and

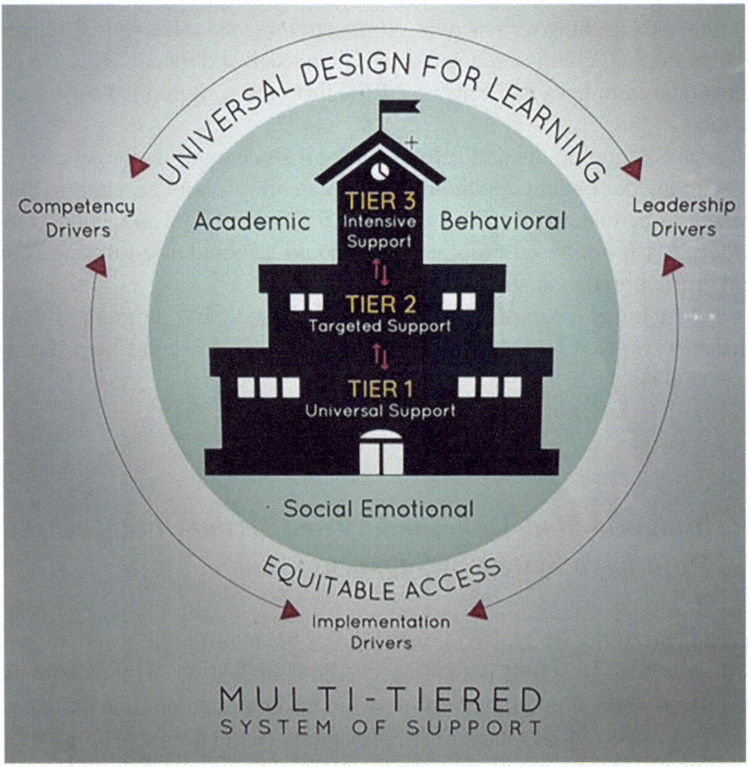

Fig. 6.2 Multitiered system of support (Massachusetts Department of Elementary and Secondary Education, 2023)

seen as goals to achieve. While the students in each tier require different levels of instruction, including the regular classroom, small-group instruction in the classroom may be designed for specific tiers. Key elements of MTSS are the administration of screening surveys or tests at least three times a year, regular probes to monitor progress, and regular staff conferencing to review data and strategized lesson plans.

MTSS became the overarching referent for frameworks designed to proactively target behavioral and academic challenges with a focus on emphasizing a tiered continuum of evidence-based practices within the context of prevention science and implementation research (Freeman et al., 2016). The goal of MTSS is to create a student-centered, formative framework that uses preventative problem-solving and evidence-based practices to address difficulties among students (Hunter et al., 2015). MTSS has emerged as the single best effort to provide a preventative, decision-making, problem-solving, evidence-based framework that addresses the interconnectedness of academic and behavioral difficulties (Nelson et al., 2004).

There is an extensive literature demonstrating the effectiveness of MTSS programs, particularly for addressing the academic and behavioral needs of diverse student bodies (see Berkeley et al., 2008; Landers et al., 2012). According to Eagle et al. (2014), "increasing attention has been placed on the need for an integrated model that braids initiatives for academic, behavioral and social-emotional needs into a single Multi-Tiered System of Support (MTSS)." Ten years later, this has happened.

Most of the BridgeUp schools created specific "Tier 2" classes on the school campus. For students who needed more serious mental health supports, such as intervention for self-harming behaviors, protocols with established mental health partners set the referral parameters. These "Tier 3" students were then referred to a mental health partner such as Menninger.

US national studies report that 15–20% of students need additional supports (What is PBIS?, n.d.). Since most mental illnesses emerge before age 14 (Kessler et al., 2005), it is crucial to identify additional supports for these students early on. During the last 5 years of the BridgeUp project, approximately 6% of the students in the BridgeUp cohort needed a referral for additional supports, such as peer or group counseling, and approximately 4% of the students needed more serious mental health supports. Thus, on average, the BridgeUp student population needing additional mental health supports was lower overall than for the US population.

For many, there is not a diagnosable mental illness in need of treatment. Rather, mental health issues arise for adolescents due to a number of nonmedical reasons, including social or relational family conflicts or illness. Since a majority of the BridgeUp students were disadvantaged (an average of 79%), many experienced mental health challenges due to changes in family structure or place of residence, including some of the students becoming orphans due to having incarcerated parents. During the pandemic, 54% of students surveyed in a BridgeUp charter school were responsible for caring for a family member (Personal Communication, Ryan Villarreal, 2021).

Connection to caring adults was built into the BridgeUp model with the SEL instruction, so trust could build over time with students. Therefore, when the need for support occurred, the adult could help facilitate the process for the student quickly. A mental health referral protocol identified what kind of supports would best serve the students. Accommodations or supports could be accessed early and often when a student requested help. Similarly, if others such as a teacher, administrator, or parent noticed that a student seemed to be suffering alone, they could request support on behalf of the student.

This was the case with Amy, an 11th grader from a BridgeUp school (see Fig. 6.3). She had been a part of the BridgeUp program since she was in eighth grade, developing trusted connections with the BridgeUp codirectors. The codirectors applied for a seed grant from BridgeUp to establish mentoring discussion groups for adolescents who needed a regular, safe space to share their experiences and challenges with their peers. In partnership with a local church, 50 students were invited to sign up, attend, and become a part of the weekly groups. Amy was one of those students, and her story is representative of the value of student and teacher relationships that result from a strong, school-based prevention program integrated throughout the school day, over a period of years (See Allen et al., 2021).

6.4.2.1 Processes for Identifying, Supporting, and Monitoring MTSS Tiers 2 and 3 Students

The processes for identifying students for additional supports varied with the school and/or school district. The procedures and protocols were not mandated by the BridgeUp model but instead deferred to the school administration. These included identification plans and screening tools reviewed by assessment teams, which gathered data to assist in making the best recommendations and referrals. Consequently, the BridgeUp cohorts presented a variety of approaches.

BridgeUp Center at The Menninger Clinic Case Report – Amy Diaz and Mirella Sales

TIER I BridgeUp Duration 8th – 12th grade
Suburban Charter School

Amy attended a BridgeUp Charter school located in a highly diverse, mostly low-income, suburban Houston neighborhood. Since she was part of the BridgeUp project from its inception, she developed trusted connections with the BridgeUp co-directors, one of whom was Mirella Sales. Mirella invited Amy to participate in a year-long after-school mentoring group, where Amy found a sense of belonging and developed authentic and meaningful friendships with other students and adults.

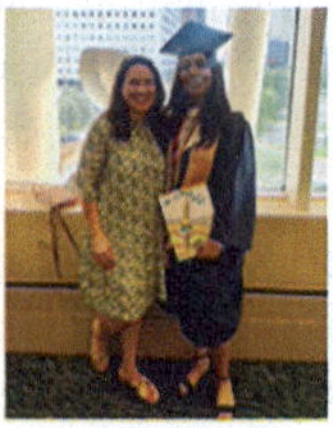

When Mirella discovered that Amy had the potential to attend a prestigious college, she encouraged her to apply. Upon acceptance to the University of Chicago, Amy was conflicted about attending and leaving her traditional Hispanic family, as she would be the first one to leave home and move away for college.

Mirella escorted her to the campus, and Amy says the trip was a life-changing experience. Amy is now a rising junior, with aspirations of becoming a neuroscientist.

Fig. 6.3 BridgeUp Center at The Menninger Clinic Case Report—Amy Diaz and Mirella Sales. (By permission from Amy Diaz, Mirella Sales and The Menninger Clinic)

Despite these variations, the Patient Health Questionnaire-9 (PHQ-9) (APA, n.d.) and the Pediatric System Checklist (PSC-17) (Massachusetts General Hospital: Psychiatry, n.d.) are screening tool examples used in the BridgeUp schools (See also, Trafalis et al., 2021). A shared decision-making approach was used in the BridgeUp schools for appropriate referrals. A mental health professional was part of that team, which discussed the best treatment and provider referral for the students.

The most frequent process for supporting Tier 2 BridgeUp students was small-group sessions, typically held at the school. These usually comprised an average of five students and facilitated by trained classroom teachers, school counselors, or community agency specialists. The session length of time as well as the frequency varied among the different schools. Sometimes, they met in the homeroom period or after school for specific programming.

Since there was a formal memorandum of understanding between the school and a mental health provider, Tier 3 BridgeUp students were referred to the designated partner, which typically included a federally qualified health center, private mental health provider, or The Menninger Clinic. The first BridgeUp Tier 3 student, Jo Jo, was an eighth-grade student at a large suburban middle school (see Fig. 6.4). Despite her outward appearance, she struggled internally. Because of the BridgeUp project that was just implemented in her school, the mental health referral team made the recommendation that Jo Jo go to Menninger for a mental health assessment. As reported in a later chapter in this volume, there are many barriers to care for adolescents (See for example, AHRQ, 2023). Although Jo Jo experienced several barriers to seeking treatment, she eventually went to Menninger.

Monitoring Tiers 2 and 3 BridgeUp students for follow-up was a challenging task for all of the schools. Usually, a small team would follow up with the

BridgeUp Center at The Menninger Clinic Case Report – Jo Jo Garcia

TIER III BridgeUp Duration 8th – 12th grade
Suburban Large Public School District

Jolianna "Jo Jo" Garcia is an 18-year-old Hispanic female adolescent completing her senior year in high school. At age 13, she attended a suburban middle school in a predominantly Hispanic area of Houston, where she was part of the inaugural BridgeUp project. Jo Jo was a member of the junior national honor society, played viola in the orchestra, excelled on the volleyball team, and maintained straight A's. At first glance, one might presume she was destined to become a high school valedictorian. However, inwardly, Jo Jo struggled with depression, self-doubt, low self-confidence, and self-harm.

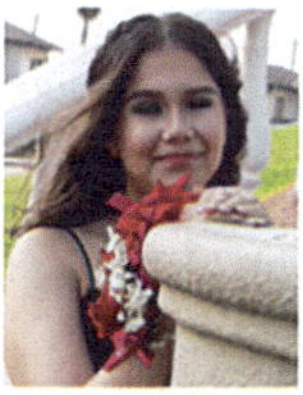

The school counselor raised concerns about Jo Jo's well-being. Because of the BridgeUp project, she was referred to Menninger for a mental health assessment. Jo Jo was subsequently admitted to the inpatient Adolescent Treatment Program (ATP) for two weeks, followed by six weeks of intensive outpatient care. Upon returning to school after nearly two months, she anticipated resuming her previous activities. However, she was met with meanness and bullying from her volleyball teammates. Despite interventions from counselors, principals, teachers, and her mother, the mistreatment persisted.

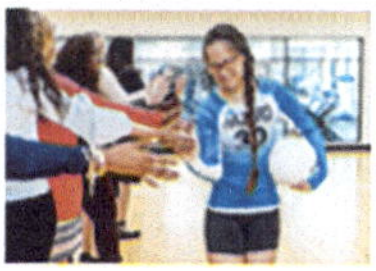

Five years later, Jo Jo is a member of the National Honor Society and preparing to attend college next year. She has experienced significant personal growth driven by her aspiration to effect positive change in the world. Jo Jo now aims to become an advocate for adolescent girls grappling with mental health issues. She has returned to Menninger's ATP campus to address current residents, offering them reassurance and hope for the future.

Fig. 6.4 BridgeUp Center at The Menninger Clinic Case Report—Jo Jo Garcia. (By permission from Jo Jo Lovos Garcia, Licette Lovos and The Menninger Clinic)

effectiveness of the early interventions, which was easier with Tier 2 students since they were on campus, with some students opting to continue with the groups and become peer counselors. Because the Tier 3 students were off campus for more intensive supports and treatment, follow-up proved to be more difficult and is an area for improvement in the future. This was especially true regarding the provider evaluations and the lack of follow-up. This was alleviated somewhat by the students themselves who felt connected with the school and provided their own follow-up.

6.4.2.2 Processes and Protocol Examples for Early Intervention Referral

As mentioned above, each school developed customized Tier 2 and 3 referral programs. The example in Table 6.1 is a brief example of how a Texas school district, with approximately 17,000 students, developed, trained, and implemented the programs, curricula, and referral criteria. Mental health providers were selected at the beginning of the school year (BridgeUp at Menninger, 2022b).

Tier 2 students were referred based on a customized *Panorama* survey (Panorama Education, n.d.). They received an array of in-school Tier 2 programming. Students in Tier 1 or Tier 2 who demonstrated the need for more intensive supports could be referred to Tier 3. A shared decision-making team determined the best external mental health provider for referral for the individual student.

Table 6.1 BridgeUp at Menninger example of Tier 1, 2, and 3 programs and referral to services

Tier	Target student group	Programs, curricula	Mental health assessment, behavioral health services
Tier 1	All students (universal)	7 mindsets curriculum (staff professional development and weekly explicit instruction for students)	
Tier 2	1. Students with demonstrated deficits in SEL 2. Students with needs in mental health areas (self-injury, grief, anxiety)	Program Why Try Resilience for Youth The Anxiety Workbook for Teens Stopping the Pain	Data from panorama survey measuring student SEL competency
Tier 3	Students with intense mental health or behavioral needs requiring ongoing, individual intervention		Referral to pre-authorized mental health providers, including A private provider A county service provider The Menninger Clinic

6.4.3 BridgeUp Model's Third Framework: Collective Impact[1]

The third framework of the BridgeUp model is an evidence-based framework utilizing the *collective impact* (CI) approach (Kania & Kramer, 2011). These authors describe the five conditions that are necessary for successful collaborative results, including a backbone support organization, a common agenda, shared measurement systems, mutually reinforcing activities, and continuous communication.

The lead BridgeUp director's school or organization served as the backbone agency for each grant. Shared metrics were developed by the BridgeUp leadership team, with input from the Advisory Committee. In addition, all of the schools created their own measurement systems to track students by using tools, such as PowerSchool, formerly known as Kickboard (PowerSchool, n.d.). These tools helped schools enhance their school culture and positive well-being of the whole child/adolescent by managing outcomes from SEL and MTSS.

The BridgeUp RFP helped to frame the reinforcing activities in a way that served as a template, with intentional flexibility and adaptability built-in so that the model worked across varying dimensions. These included school size, culture, and diversity, among other categories that included inner-city and suburban, under-resourced, and more affluent school districts.

Continuous communication was achieved with the partners through regular check-in meetings with the BridgeUp lead. One BridgeUp school designated four teachers in a school with about 800 students to be "SEL ambassadors," which helped to structure the communication pathways across the school.

Public health research and interventions typically work across many disciplines, and collaboration with multisectoral partners is necessary to achieve system change. The three core, interconnected systems included multiple partners within the adolescent mental health, public health, and school health systems, and all played vital roles in implementing the system change with the BridgeUp model (see, e.g., Hunter & Mpofu, 2022). Thus, all BridgeUp grants required multisectoral collaboration structured with the CI requirements. Overall, this process worked smoothly, even when there were more than three or four organizations per cohort. Some school districts had as many as 10 or 12 partners.

6.4.3.1 Video: Cherié Spencer, on Amplifying Collaboration (2019)

One of the long-term BridgeUp grantees was the Galveston Independent School District, located in Galveston Texas, just 50 miles from Houston. Their BridgeUp Director, Cherié Spencer, speaks in this video (Video 6.1) about the benefits of collaboration and how it has dramatically improved what they were able to do for adolescent mental health in their school district (Personal Communication, Cherié Spencer, 2019).

[1] More detail about collective impact is included in the preceding chapter.

6.4.3.2 The BridgeUp Impact Network

The BridgeUp leadership convened all of the grant projects quarterly, in what was called the BridgeUp Impact Network. In partnership with the University of Houston's All Kids Alliance, the Impact Network created a shared learning community and gave guidance to each grant partner throughout the academic year. The BridgeUp Impact Network was modeled on a similar approach employed by the StriveTogether Network, with which a member (RW) of our leadership team was familiar with implementing. The StriveTogether approach, in turn, was based on the *Collaborative Model for Achieving Breathrough Improvement* designed by the Institute for Healthcare Improvement (2003). The Impact Network participants included the grant lead organizations, including school districts and nonprofit organizations, and all supplementary, collaborative agencies providing curriculum support, student or teacher support, or mental health services. There was an average of 40 organizations participating in the BridgeUp Impact Network each year. The quarterly convenings of the BridgeUp cohort became increasingly formalized and strategic over time, resulting in improvement of the model implementation.

Another reason that the CI approach worked well was because of shared accountability. All of the BridgeUp schools and organizations were serving vulnerable adolescents, especially those disadvantaged and living in underserved communities. The grant required equal status among the partners and, therefore, equal status in shared accountability. The Impact Network meetings served as an opportunity for the different cohorts to share challenges and successes, despite each having different approaches to achieving improved adolescent mental health with the same BridgeUp model.

To foster shared accountability, BridgeUp introduced Magic Grants recipients to visualizing tools, including theory of change (ToC), logic models (LM), and rapid cycle improvement (RCI). These approaches and strategies were covered in the previous chapter, so the next section will give examples of how these were used with the BridgeUp model.

6.4.3.3 Theory of Change[2] Implementation

To advance its theory of change, each grant partnership described how it would engage teachers and students when offering SEL programming (Tier 1) and MTSS services (Tiers 2 and 3) for students who needed early interventions through small-group consultations or targeted, individual therapy. Additionally, the partnerships declared the "changes" or outcomes that their efforts were intended to produce. Here, they were encouraged to think in relatively short time frames and to describe the desired changes in learning and behavior.

[2] More detail about theory of change is included in the preceding chapter.

There are many ways to model a theory of change. A worksheet approach, such as the one displayed here in Fig. 6.5, can guide a provider through the steps. Note that some worksheets use "theory of change" to describe generic challenges, activities or resources, short-term change processes, and impacts, which they couple with a "theory of action" in which each generic element (on the left) is specified in detail (on the right). This is the tool that was offered to the BridgeUp partnerships.

Once a partnership created an explicated theory of change, they were coached and participated in constructing a logic model.

6.4.3.4 Logic Models[3]

Bridge Up partnerships constructed logic models to translate their theories of change into a logical and measurable flow of events. The purpose of this exercise was to prompt members to specifically state the expected outcomes at each stage in

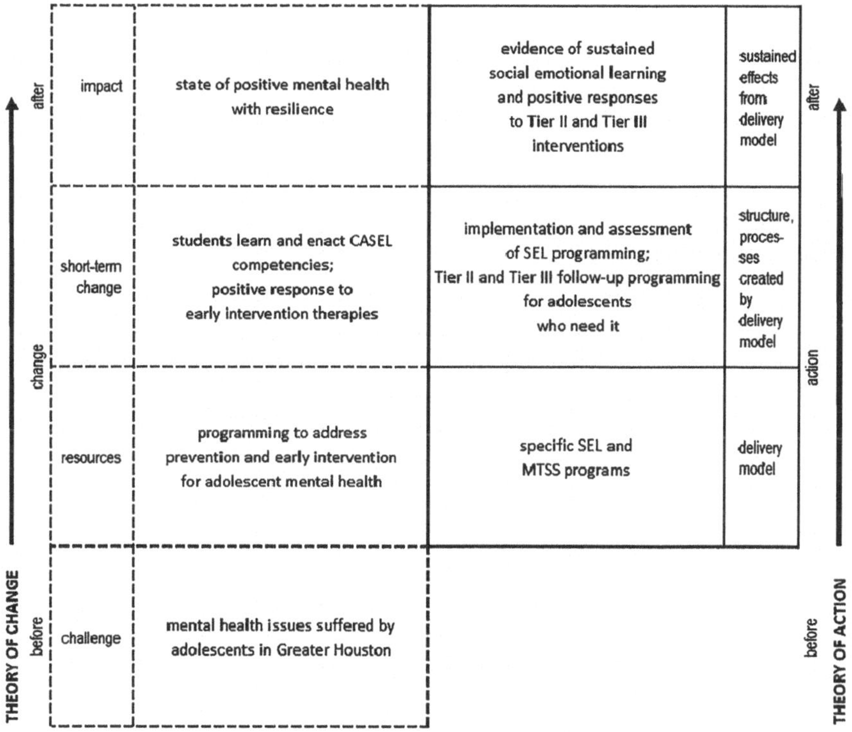

Fig. 6.5 BridgeUp theory of change worksheet. (By Permission from All Kids Alliance, University of Houston and The Menninger Clinic)

[3] More detail about logic models is included in the preceding chapter.

the logical sequence and to tell them if they were on a path to success (Fig. 6.6). Outcomes of the BridgeUp model were based on the SEL outcomes that align with Durlak et al. (2015). These included SEL competencies learned, improved discipline, mental health and well-being and academic performance outcomes.

Over the course of the six-year grant cycles, numerous implementation changes and adjustments were made from the original concept. This is actually how system change should work.

6.4.3.5 Rapid Cycle Improvement

In the BridgeUp model, specifying and measuring outputs is prerequisite to tracking outcomes. Without data on outputs, data on outcomes would have little or no meaning. And even if desired outcomes showed improvement, there could be little assurance about the degree to which positive change could be attributed to a cohort's programming. In this way, rapid cycle improvement involves short-cycle gauges of effectiveness such that regular corrections can be made in real time while programs are being implemented.

Measuring improvement requires an appeal to the data collected. Structuring and collecting data are often left out of budgets but are critical to sustainable programming. Traditionally, funding for nonprofit organizations requires a midyear and an

LOGIC MODEL: *Rapid Cycle Continuous Improvement*			**defining success**		
EFFORTS		>	EFFECTS		
Processes		>	Short-Term ⟶	**Outcomes** ⟶	Long-Term
What are the main **Activities** you are employing?	What will be the **Outputs** of your activities?	>	What will **Learning** look like?	What **Behavior Change** will take place?	What **Impact** will that learning and behavior change have?
students are exposed to Tier I, Tier II, and Tier III programming	*students are present during Tier I, Tier II, and/or Tier III activities* *students are actively engaged during these activities* *teachers/counselors therapists undertake activities effectively, with fidelity to program standards*	> > > > >	*students learn social emotional language* *students gain self-awareness around social emotional states of mind*	*students interact using the language of social emotional learning* *students demonstrate self-control and empathy*	*students demonstrate long-term resilience with or without support*

Fig. 6.6 Logic model for BridgeUp Magic Grants and rapid cycle improvement: defining success. (By Permission from All Kids Alliance, University of Houston and The Menninger Clinic)

annual evaluation of variables that are not always "improvement" related. Despite funders providing evaluation templates for their desired outcomes, there are still consistent challenges, not to mention missed opportunities. This typical kind of evaluation can be called a "summative" or "conclusive evaluation."

BridgeUp used a "formative" or "developmental evaluation"[4] which was adapted from a practice imbedded in the StriveTogether (2024) collective impact framework. In addition to an annual summative evaluation, each BridgeUp partnership was required to complete an ongoing developmental evaluation, using the indicator system in their logic model to collect data on a regular basis. Every 4–6 weeks, an accountability group visited each program and reviewed the accumulated data. This provided an outside view of progress toward intended outcomes and assistance in problem-solving as needed. A focus on the data is maintained with reference to possible causal links which works well with systems change initiatives (See for example, FSG: Reimagining Social Change, 2016). This group has knowledge of the success and failures of other programs allowing for cross-fertilization of solutions and ideas.

The use of the rapid cycle improvement process is an essential process that drives a robust collective impact framework and allows an organization to monitor its program, clarify and reframe the logic, and gauge the effect of its programming in a realistic time frame.

6.5 BridgeUp Model Implementation

Using implementation science (Bauer & Kirchner, 2020), the BridgeUp model implementation occurred during the 2016–2022 academic years. The first half of the implementation period included a *Pilot Phase I* with progressive additional enhancements annually. The second half of the implementation period, from 2019 to 2022, included a focus on strategic scalability and sustainability. This *Scalability and Sustainability Phase II* was guided by a formal strategic plan that included refined implementation approaches, enhanced program evaluation, capacity building for scalability, sustainability, and key performance indicators (KPIs) for the BridgeUp Center.

Initially, a funding distribution plan was developed to cover the entire 6-year period. This included a planned, incremental increase of funding through the end of the Pilot Phase I. The intent was to cast the net wide enough to test the model with different schools, school districts, and other variables, such as after-school or in-school implementation. The peak of the funding occurred during the end of the Pilot Phase I and began decreasing over the remaining 3-year period with the Scalability and Sustainability Phase II.

Throughout the duration of the project, the BridgeUp Impact Network group met in person and remotely when the schools were closed due to COVID-19. The proliferation of the model and the lessons learned from each cohort were shared across the greater Houston area, through many presentations and regional conferences.

[4] Developmental evaluation refers to collecting and analyzing data to inform decision making during the implementation process. (See FSG: Reimagining Social Change, (2016).

6.6 Model Implementation: Pilot Phase I

2016–2019 Academic Years

The Pilot Phase I began with the 2016–2017 academic year, which included 30 partnerships between 28 schools, after-school programs, nonprofits including mental health partners, and one school district. All of the programs were bound together by BridgeUp commitments to the BridgeUp five principles and themes of integration and equity.

By the end of the BridgeUp program in 2022, only schoolwide programs were funded, with preference for the model to be implemented district-wide.

6.6.1 Phase I Strategic Planning

Strategic planning was a critical factor for the BridgeUp outcomes. The focus for the beginning of the project included hiring a leadership team and educating the Menninger leadership team about BridgeUp. There were three overarching and strategic goals during the 3-year pilot phase. The 11 objectives for the 3 goals were enhanced each year, beginning with choosing the inaugural collaborative grant cohorts of schools and nonprofit organizations.

- The first goal was to implement, monitor, and refine the model and evaluation metrics as a measurable tool for innovation and system change regarding adolescent mental health and well-being. Each year, the process became more efficient and easier to implement, with an expanded reach from 1495 students the first year to 8250 the second year. Additionally, 670 teachers, administrators, and parents were trained in SEL. The total number of students reached during the pilot phase was 18,606.
- The second goal was to convene the quarterly Impact Network, mentioned earlier in this chapter. The purpose of the Impact Network was for all BridgeUp partners to meet as a shared learning community and to provide support to their peer colleagues. Professional learning topics, such as appropriate screening tools, rapid cycle improvement, and evaluation metrics, were always a part of the convenings, led by the BridgeUp leadership team. The overall collective impact "backbone" role was filled by BridgeUp.
- A third goal was for Menninger to contribute to the mental health and well-being of adolescents in the larger community. This included numerous community engagement opportunities, such as asking Menninger clinicians to help the inaugural grantees. For example, one of the Menninger psychologists helped to produce bilingual parent engagement mental health videos for a BridgeUp school district. Another example included multiple media opportunities to discuss adolescent mental health challenges and possible solutions. BridgeUp school leaders and adolescents had the opportunity to participate in these numerous events.

6.6.2 *The New BridgeUp Model*

The full BridgeUp model rolled out during the 2016–2017 academic year. The mental health literacy part of the model was successfully implemented with CASEL's SEL prevention framework in mostly after-school programs during the first year. The second framework of the model included a MTSS mental health referral system that was customized by each partner. This resulted in 499 or 33% of the students referred to one of the mental health partners for additional mental health supports. This percentage was much higher than the national average of 20%. All of the inaugural grants represented the most vulnerable adolescents in low performing and/or underserved geographic areas and school. For example, one partner was working with the lowest performing school in Texas, which created multiple challenges for implementation and BridgeUp project retention. However, after only one semester with the BridgeUp funding, significant progress was demonstrated (See Mellon, 2016 for a feature story on this partner). The innovation with this school included funding a nonprofit to provide wraparound services for students like "Kevin," in Box 6.4.

The third part of the model regarding collective impact was achieved with 58 schools, nonprofits, and mental health organizations participating in the inaugural year.

On a separate note, for the pilot rollout, several different BridgeUp types of programs were implemented, including a *model* grant, with the specific task of piloting and implementing the full BridgeUp model. A smaller *innovation* grant offered an

Box 6.4: A Successful Example of High School Wraparound Services
When Kevin was identified by the nonprofit working with the lowest performing school in Texas, he was in the 10th grade and his average attendance was a staggering 63%. Kevin had accumulated more than 30 behavioral referrals to an alternative school. Everyone labeled Kevin as a lost cause and no one sought to understand the root his the problems. Kevin lived in a hostile home environment with five other siblings. Despite both of his parents working, their combined income was less than $35,000 per year. There were numerous interventions by the schools, which were ineffective.

The nonprofit was able to assess Kevin's assets and needs and linked him to mentorship, health services, workforce development, and social services. A personalized bundle of services was made available to address the interdependencies of educational, social, and healthcare needs.

After participating in these programs, Kevin's school attendance improved to 90%, with only three behavioral referrals and improved academic performance. This enabled Kevin to graduate from high school and begin his studies at Houston Baptist University.

opportunity that was similar to a planning grant. Both were successful and, in several cases, an innovation grant became a model grant the following year.

6.6.3 Adaptations of the Model

Three important adaptations were offered during the pilot phase. The first variation preferred that schools (and not nonprofits) serve as fiscal agents and grant leads for the partnership. With the experience from the disruption resulting from Hurricane Harvey (Box 6.5), the BridgeUp leadership team discovered the difficulty for external nonprofit organizations serving as the grant leads. Multilayered new initiatives need school authority (and not external organizations) to make decisions on behalf of the school, especially in times of disruption.

The second adaptation concerned the SEL intervention to build skills for mental health literacy, which is the first part of the BridgeUp model. CASEL-based SEL programs were implemented in schools at a much faster rate than before ESSA was active across the USA in 2017. As SEL uptake increased across the country, more research was published. BridgeUp subsequently used this research to make evidence-based adjustments for the grant requirements . One significant finding recommended that SEL be integrated (a) schoolwide and (b) throughout all school day classes and not just in homeroom or after school. The grant guidelines were adjusted to accommodate this change in the model.

The third important finding recommended SEL training for the teachers and staff since it was revealed that they needed social and emotional learning training just like the students. Eventually, best practice included implementing the model in most classes, schoolwide, with no after-school programs. A key organization from the Houston Theater district was one of the key BridgeUp partners during this pilot phase. They designed SEL classes to be taught through the lens of dramatic arts, including in science class. This was one of the students' favorite approaches to SEL throughout the duration of the BridgeUp project.

Box 6.5: Example of School Disruptions

During the second pilot year, Hurricane Harvey arrived at the beginning of a new school semester, devastating the Texas Gulf Coast area with massive flooding, canceling schools, and disrupting more than one million public school students (ABC News, 2017). After Harvey, the RFP requirements were changed to ensure that schools acted as fiscal agents and grant leads. This policy worked well when COVID-19 happened a few years later. Nonprofits and mental health providers remained as collaborative partners, which enabled the intervention to work seamlessly, especially for the integration of MTSS.

6.6.4 A Note About Innovation

Frieden (2014) writes about the six components necessary for effective public health program implementation. Similar to entrepreneurial start-ups, innovation can be a core component in adolescent mental health system change. During COVID-19, there were many examples of innovation in adolescent mental health, such as with telepsychiatry for adults and adolescents (Prisco et al., 2020).

Entrepreneurial start-ups have five stages of growth development and usually reach success during Stage 3 (Churchill & Lewis, 1983). The research shows that when entrepreneurs begin a new business, it usually takes 2–3 years to become stable and successful (Ding, 2023). With the case of the BridgeUp implementation, the successful pilot phase was completed in 3.5 years.

6.7 Model Implementation: Scalability and Sustainability Phase II

2019–2022 Academic Years

Following the BridgeUp Pilot Phase I was the Scalability and Sustainability Phase II, which included strategic planning; expanded shared measurement; improved theory of change (ToC), logic models (LM), and rapid cycle improvement (RCI); and the development of scalability and sustainability implementation plans. Although positive outcomes were experienced after the first academic semester, it took time to test and continuously adapt the model. Therein lies the conundrum when it comes to innovation. The obvious factor was that in 2015, there was limited evidence-based research to support a *new* AMH model, although there was evidence to support and inform each of the three frameworks that comprised the model. Similar to the healthcare entrepreneur start-ups, a formal, more strategic approach, with enhanced standardization and specific metrics, was required. Therefore, midway through the project, the BridgeUp leadership team collaborated once again with the University of Houston's All Kids Alliance to create an actionable, data-driven, 3-year strategic plan.

6.7.1 Phase II Strategic Planning

A multidisciplinary Strategic Planning Task Force included leaders from Menninger and the BridgeUp community. During the 9-month planning sessions, multiple interviews with key stakeholders were conducted, with formal meetings held monthly. Based on these findings and the evaluation data from Phase I, a final strategic planning document was completed. The plan included SMART goals[5] and

[5]The mnemonic acronym SMART stands for specific, measurable, achievable, relevant, and time-bound.

corresponding annual metrics, which rolled out at the beginning of the 2019–2020 academic year. BridgeUp produced a 3-year strategic plan that was a vital communication tool internally and externally (BridgeUp at Menninger, 2019). This summary statement captured the lessons learned from the Pilot Phase I implementation and helped to structure the Scalability and Sustainability Phase II, as follows:

> We believe that our commitment to children and youth requires us to be honest and transparent so that our relationships are anchored in trust. We also believe that good stewardship of the resources with which we are entrusted obligates us to pursue continuous improvement in the ways we serve and empower children and youth. BridgeUp wedded these two commitments – to transparency and continuous improvement – by creating a Strategic Plan that guides our work through its goals, strategies, and key performance indicators.

This working strategic plan included 9 goals with 27 strategies organized with annual outcomes and KPIs. Table 6.2 represents the progress at the end of the BridgeUp program (BridgeUp at Menninger, 2019). As the year over year results demonstrate, the strategic plan goals were mostly achieved as originally envisioned, although COVID-19 restricted progress on achieving the growth Goals 6 and 7 and the BridgeUp funding was not renewed for Goal 3, indicated with an asterisk.

Table 6.2 A 3-year strategic plan

BridgeUp 2020 - 2022			
Year 1	**Year 2**	**Year 3**	**Strategic Goals**
July 2019 – 2020	**July 2020 – 2021**	**July 2021 – 2022**	
Goal 1	**Goal 1**	**Goal 1**	Sustain Current BridgeUp Partnerships
Goal 2	**Goal 2**	**Goal 2**	Develop BridgeUp Evaluation Systems
Goal 3	**Goal 3**	***Goal 3**	Secure BridgeUp Funding Through FY2029
Goal 4	**Goal 4**	**Goal 4**	Specify Oversight and Accountability
Goal 5	**Goal 5**	**Goal 5**	Move to Funding Only School-Wide Programs
Goal 6	***Goal 6**	***Goal 6**	Introduce BridgeUp Statewide
Goal 7	***Goal 7**	***Goal 7**	Introduce BridgeUp Nationally to Hospital Systems
Goal 8	**Goal 8**	**Goal 8**	Spread Awareness of Model Across Regional ISDs
Goal 9	**Goal 9**	**Goal 9**	Create Toolkit for Replicability and Scalability

Used by permission from The Menninger Clinic

6.7.1.1 Phase II Strategic Plan: Sustainability, Scalability, Replicability, and Evaluation

The strategic plan included an expanded ToC, LM, and RCI, which helped the BridgeUp partnerships determine what was and was not working earlier and with more specificity. Often with external funding to schools, programs can become one-offs because there is not a strategic commitment to attend to extending the life of the program. Therefore, of special interest during Phase II was how best to scale and sustain the model in schools and school districts beyond the life of the BridgeUp Center. What the Phase II revealed was that the program worked best when integrated into the school day and within the school administrative procedures. This coupled with enhanced evaluation methods rounded out the plan, as follows in Box 6.6 (BridgeUp at Menninger, 2019).

Box 6.6: Strategic Plan: Sustainability, Scalability, Replicability, and Evaluation (BridgeUp at Menninger, 2019)

1. Sustainability
   - Provide capacity building to sustain current BridgeUp programs.
   - Secure ongoing matched funding for the partnerships in the schools.
   - Secure ongoing BridgeUp funding at the end of the program.
2. Scalability and replicability
   - Scale programs school- and district-wide.
   - Disseminate the BridgeUp model regionally, statewide, and nationally.
   - Create a BridgeUp toolkit for replicability and scalability.
3. Evaluation
   - Establish metrics for a BridgeUp growth strategy.
   - Develop BridgeUp program evaluation systems that analyze students' specific outcomes from the partners' SEL programs. SEL competencies help to prepare young people to succeed in college, work, family, and society.
   - Since research shows that improving SEL competencies creates positive outcomes, listed below, there was motivation to enhance the measurement of these competencies (Denham, 2015).
     - Self-awareness
     - Self-management
     - Social awareness
     - Relationship skills
     - Responsible decision-making
   - Refine the ToC, LM, and RCI processes and metrics for all partners to increase effectiveness.

Part of the reasons for success of the BridgeUp model included building capacity within current BridgeUp partnerships. Specifically, the goal was for them to prepare accordingly for model sustainability when the BridgeUp initiative ended in 2022. BridgeUp worked with the Rice University's Center for Philanthropy and Nonprofit Leadership to assist in this effort by meeting one-on-one with each of the BridgeUp partnerships. Each partnership created a funding plan that included a complete budget (with actual and in-kind costs) and gaps in resources, along with a presentation and a case for support to provide internally to their School Boards or externally to other funders.

By implementing intentional capacity building throughout the Sustainability Phase, BridgeUp ensured that all partners were in a strong position to scale and sustain their programs. Additionally, the BridgeUp model could be sustained in schools independently without the funding and an external backbone agency. The BridgeUp toolkit is available online for those interested in learning more (BridgeUp at Menninger, 2022a). Ultimately, through scalability and sustainability, more students, like the eighth grader from a BridgeUp school writing in her journal (image captured in Fig. 6.7), would be reached at new schools and districts into the future.

6.8 Evaluation Overview

BridgeUp designed and implemented a multifaceted evaluation, which included the (1) the Magic Grants evaluation requirements and (2) the BridgeUp evaluation requirements. From the inception of the project, continuous outcomes were tracked and monitored becoming increasingly robust for the Magic Grants over time. The evaluation requirements for the Magic Grants partners and for the BridgeUp Center are listed below. This section presents descriptions and examples of the quantitative and qualitative data used for the 46 interventions for the 6-year implementation of the BridgeUp model.

The program evaluations were decentralized to individual schools and districts. This served as an important lesson in terms of promoting long-term sustainability.

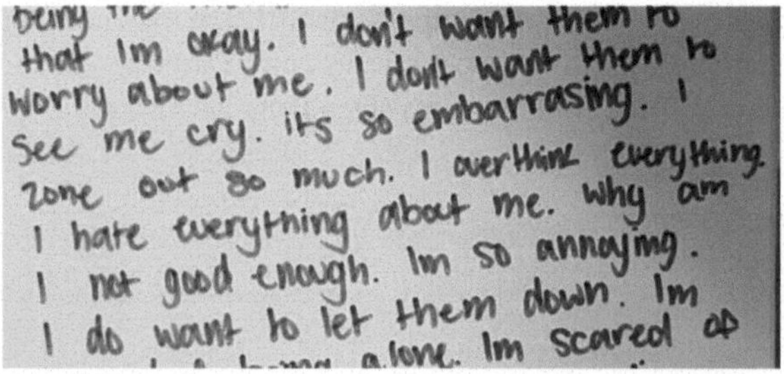
that Im okay. I don't want them to
worry about me. I don't want them to
see me cry. its so embarrasing. I
zone out so much. I overthink everything.
I hate everything about me. why am
I not good enough. Im so annoying.
I do want to let them down. Im

Fig. 6.7 BridgeUp school. SEL Journal Excerpt. School Year FY2021–2022. (By permission from The Menninger Clinic)

1. The Magic Grants evaluation requirements included:
   (a) Midyear and Annual Program Evaluation
   (b) Midyear and Annual BridgeUp Mixed Method Evaluation Report
   (c) BridgeUp Special Topic Surveys
   (d) Rapid Cycle Improvement Evaluation (2018–2022)
   (e) Impact Network Surveys

Evaluation Metrics

There was a wide assortment of evaluation metrics used by the schools and nonprofits, covering academics, attendance, behavior, SEL, SEL self-assessment, and school culture. Based on the SEL literature (see Durlak et al., 2011, 2015), SEL outcomes measured by all grantees included

(i) Enhanced SEL Skills and Competencies
(ii) Reduced disciplinary infractions and school suspensions
(iii) Positive effects regarding improved mental health and well-being
(iv) Improved Academic Performance

An example of metrics and instruments that one grants partner used is presented in Table 6.3.

Over time, the SEL metrics continued to improve. Prior to COVID-19, the following outcomes (Denham, 2015) were observed: increased SEL competencies, decreased disciplinary infractions, significant decrease in suicide risk, and an increase in math and reading scores.

One of the most important outcomes during the entire BridgeUp project was providing additional mental health supports and treatment to 6232 underserved adolescents. Most of these students were disadvantaged and did not have access to care, including primary care or mental health.

Table 6.3 Examples of evaluation metrics adopted and tracked by BridgeUp schools

Academics	**Attendance**	**Behavior**
Benchmark assessments	Daily rate	Office discipline referrals
STAAR algebra/English	Average daily rate	After-school detention
Grade promotion		In-school suspensions
Graduation rate		Out-of-school suspensions
Social and emotional learning	**SEL self-assessment**	**School culture**
Booth/BOSS evaluations	Panorama-teacher rating	School accountability rating
Kickboard aligned with CASEL	SSIS-teacher rating	California healthy kids survey
4th R surveys, student and teacher		
Washoe County district SEL survey		
Austin district SEL survey		
Panorama		
Choices survey/YRBS		

Source: Used by permission from The Menninger Clinic

There are many barriers to care for adolescents, including structural barriers, such as the location of the service provider. Additionally, parental perceptions about adolescent mental health problems and services are also barriers to care, according to Owens et al. (2002). These barriers were observed with the BridgeUp students and served as important lessons learned.[6]

Special Topic Surveys

Special topic surveys were conducted throughout the project within the schools and from BridgeUp. One BridgeUp survey that was conducted across all partnerships identified the top 3 supports and needs for students and teachers at the end of the academic year 2021–2022 (BridgeUp at Menninger, 2022b). Table 6.4 gives an example of a BridgeUp Student Supports and Needs Survey, which helped shape priorities for the entire group.

Referrals and tracking systems were important for each school to develop. The outcomes that were vital to the BridgeUp implementation included the numbers of Tiers 2 and 3 students reached, the causes of the referrals, and the recidivism rates. These were tracked year over year. Throughout the BridgeUp project, schools were encouraged to create their own student behavioral tracking systems and use the data to improve the BridgeUp model implementation. The schools that created these had a much more comprehensive and efficient process for following the at-risk students. Kevin's turnaround story mentioned above is an example of a school that created a comprehensive system.

Growth happened year over year, beginning with Phase I, which exceeded expectations based on the model implementation benchmarks. The Phase II growth included enhanced measurement systems, scalability, and sustainability and is represented in Table 6.5.

2. The Menninger Clinic and the HGB Foundation requirements for BridgeUp
   (a) The BridgeUp Center Community Engagement Log
   (b) The Menninger Clinic Foundation Committee Board Quarterly Reports
   (c) HGB Foundation-BridgeUp Center Key Performance Indicators Semiannually

Table 6.4 BridgeUp student supports and needs survey—June 2022

BridgeUp FY2022 student supports	BridgeUp FY2022 student needs
Emotional and mental health support	Consistency and routines
Behavioral support, especially early grades	Normalizing mental health discussions among students and in the classroom
Restorative practices	More opportunities for student voice
Academic support	SEL needs of their students
Improving students' self-efficacy and sense of belonging	Unwavering commitment to meet their holistic needs

[6] A chapter in this book (Chap. 9) is dedicated to adolescent mental health barriers to care.

(d) HGB Foundation-BridgeUp Center Midyear and Annual Reports
(e) The Menninger Clinic-BridgeUp Center Monthly Financial and Strategic Plan Reviews

At the end of the BridgeUp project, the community engagement log had reached into the millions due to the extensive multimedia interviews and press releases. Overall, the BridgeUp Impact is summarized in Table 6.6 (BridgeUp at Menninger, 2022b).

Table 6.5 Growth from Year 1 (2016–2017) and Year 6 (2021–2022)

Metric	Year 1 FY 2017–2018	Year 6 FY 2021–2022	Total 2016–2022
Number of students reached	1495	18,594	63,325
Number of students referred to tiers 2 or 3	499 (33%)	1427 (7.7%)	6232 (9.8%)
Number of students treated at Menninger	0	6	36
Number of schools participating	28	31	~164
Number of teachers, administrators, parents trained	670	1918	~6470

Source: Used by permission from The Menninger Clinic

Table 6.6 BridgeUp at Menninger mental health impacts 2015–2022

1. Maintained BridgeUp project continuity all 7 years, including hurricanes and pandemic
2. Achieved success with each part of the model: Prevention, screening, early intervention, collaboration
3. Improved outcomes for academic achievement, disciplinary infractions, SEL competencies, mental health, school connectedness
4. Enhanced Phase II—rapid cycle improvement helped to improve program efficiency and effectiveness
5. Followed a rigorous strategic planning process and met goals except growth goals (due to COVID)
6. Served as community mental health thought leader for The Menninger Clinic
7. Reached **63,325** students with BridgeUp model
8. Provided **6232** students access to mental health supports and care
9. Treated **36** BridgeUp patients at Menninger (110 students referred to Menninger)
10. Trained hundreds of schools, nonprofits, teachers, administrators, and parents
11. Partnered with Rice University, University of Houston, and Meadows Mental Health Policy Institute and numerous mental health providers
12. Supervised and trained **6** Brown fellows and **1** Brown intern
13. Provided **43** model grants and **3** seed grants
14. Received in-kind support from Menninger: Finance, IT, philanthropy, communications, and marketing
15. Raised additional BridgeUp funding with Menninger's philanthropy department
16. Matched **$9.1MM** by BridgeUp grantees for scalability
17. Sustained three independent school districts beyond BridgeUp project, reaching an estimated additional 72,000 students per year

6.9 Conclusion

This chapter highlighted the successful integrative and holistic public health approach to adolescent mental health, so that others could use the transformative model to customize system change in their schools and communities. Following the sustained challenges in schools post-pandemic, along with an adolescent health system in crisis, the learnings from the BridgeUp model provide a tested approach to a possible solution for the future. BridgeUp aligns a psychiatric health system, nonprofit organizations, and school districts to prioritize primary, secondary, and tertiary prevention, and access to treatment of mental disorders, in underserved areas. Together, more students' unmet mental health needs can be identified and addressed earlier. Providing mental health services in schools with trusted providers at low or no cost to the families significantly reduces some of the barriers to care and enhances well-being for adolescents. This helps to change the trajectory of their life course, leading to a healthy and productive adulthood, as seen with the BridgeUp students.

The ability to work closely with schools and school districts over a 6-year period allowed the BU leadership team to continuously improve the quality of the model design. By the end of year 5 (during COVID-19, academic year 2020–2021), the improvements to the model stabilized because the policies and procedures had been in place long enough for the schools to incorporate the BridgeUp model into their own administrative policies and procedures. Of the three school districts that have been sustained post-BridgeUp, two have added the BridgeUp model implementation into the annual budget for the 5-year strategic plans.

Equity, affirmation, collaboration, innovation, transformation, and integrity are the six core values for BridgeUp at Menninger. The intention of the work was to provide alternative life paths for the most vulnerable students regionally, as demonstrated with Amy, Jo Jo and Kevin in this chapter. The motivation, therefore, is to ensure that despite systemic inequalities, discrimination, poverty, and other structural societal barriers, there are opportunities to change the future for all adolescents, as well as their families, teachers, principals, schools, and communities.

This public health approach to adolescent mental health can be shared and scaled to enhance and transform adolescent mental health and forms the basis of the new *Adolescent Public Mental Health Model*. If success can happen in Texas, it can happen anywhere, since Texas ranks 46th for the highest youth mental illness prevalence and lowest for rates of youth access to care in the USA (Mental Health America, 2023).

Competing Interests

1. *The BridgeUp at Menninger study was generously funded by the David and Helen Gurley Brown Trust, BridgeUp: Mental Health at The Menninger Clinic.*
2. Patricia Gail Bray has received consultant fees from The Menninger Clinic, located in Houston, Texas.
3. Robert K. Wimpelberg has received consultant fees from The Menninger Clinic, located in Houston, Texas.

References

ABC News. (2017, August 31). More than 1 million public school students estimated to be affected by Hurricane Harvey. *ABC News*. https://abcnews.go.com/US/million-public-school-students-estimated-impacted-hurricane-harvey/story?id=49511399

Ackerman-Barger, K., Sandvold, I., Patterson, D. G., Brown, K., & Douglas-Kersellius, N. V. (2020). Leveraging collective impact to promote health equity. *Journal of Health Care for the Poor and Underserved, 31*(4S), 91–98. https://doi.org/10.1353/hpu.2020.0139

Agency for Healthcare Research and Quality (AHRQ). (2023). *2023 National Healthcare Quality and Disparities Report*. Retrieved from https://www.ahrq.gov/research/findings/nhqrdr/nhqdr23/index.html. Accessed on 10 Mar 2024.

Allen, K. A., Slaten, C. D., Arslan, G., Roffey, S., Craig, H., & Vella-Brodrick, D. A. (2021). School belonging: The importance of student and teacher relationships. In M. L. Kern & M. L. Wehmeyer (Eds.), *The Palgrave handbook of positive education*. Palgrave Macmillan. https://doi.org/10.1007/978-3-030-64537-3_21

APA. (n.d.). *Patient Health Questionnaire-9* (PHQ-9). Retrieved April 12, 2024, from https://www.apa.org/depression-guideline/patient-health-questionnaire.pdf

Bauer, M. S., & Kirchner, J. (2020). Implementation science: What is it and why should I care? *Psychiatry Research, 283*, 112376. https://doi.org/10.1016/j.psychres.2019.04.025

Berkeley, S., Bender, W. N., Peaster, L. G., & Saunders, L. (2008). Implementation of response to intervention. *Journal of Learning Disabilities, 42*(1), 85–95. https://doi.org/10.1177/0022219408326214

Black, D. L. (2021). *Essentials of social emotional learning (SEL): The complete guide for schools and practitioners* (A. S. Kaufman & N. L. Kaufman, Eds.). Wiley.

BridgeUp at Menninger. (2017). *Evaluation measures—overview* (p. 1). Unpublished Document.

BridgeUp at Menninger. (2019). *Strategic planning document*. Unpublished Document.

BridgeUp at Menninger. (2022a). *BridgeUp at Menninger: A toolkit for schools and communities supporting adolescent mental health*. https://express.adobe.com/page/b9cS5b8i6bnkY/

BridgeUp at Menninger. (2022b). *Helen Gurley Brown Foundation annual report—July 1, 2021–June 30, 2022*. Unpublished Document.

Center on Multi-Tiered System of Supports. (n.d.). *Home*. https://mtss4success.org/

Centers for Disease Control and Prevention (CDC). (2022). *The social-ecological model: A framework for prevention*. Retrieved April 9, 2024, from https://www.cdc.gov/violenceprevention/about/social-ecologicalmodel.html

Centers for Disease Control and Prevention (CDC). (2023). *Whole school, whole community, whole child (WSCC)*. Retrieved February 28, 2023, from https://www.cdc.gov/healthyschools/wscc/index.htm

Churchill, N. C., & Lewis, V. L. (1983, May). The five stages of small-business growth. *Harvard Business Review*. https://hbr.org/1983/05/the-five-stages-of-small-business-growth

Collaborative for Academic, Social and Emotional Learning. (2021, June). *The CASEL guide to schoolwide SEL essentials: A printable compilation of key activities and tools for school team*. CASEL – Guide to Schoolwide SEL. https://schoolguide.casel.org/uploads/sites/2/2019/09/2021.6.15_School-Guide-Essentials.pdf

Collaborative for Academic, Social and Emotional Learning. (n.d.-a). https://casel.org/

Collaborative for Academic, Social and Emotional Learning. (n.d.-b). *Our history*. CASEL. Retrieved September 18, 2023, from https://casel.org/about-us/our-history/

Collaborative for Academic, Social and Emotional Learning. (n.d.-c). *SEL and mental health – CASEL*. CASEL. Retrieved January 24, 2024, from https://casel.org/fundamentals-of-sel/how-does-sel-support-your-priorities/sel-and-mental-health/

Collective Impact Forum. (2022, April 14). *What is collective impact*. Retrieved November 13, 2023, from https://collectiveimpactforum.org/what-is-collective-impact/

Dahlberg, L. L., & Krug, E. G. (2002). Violence: A global public health problem. In E. Krug, L. L. Dahlberg, J. A. Mercy, A. B. Zwi, & R. Lozano (Eds.), *World report on violence and health* (pp. 1–21). World Health Organization.

Denham, S. A. (2015). Assessment of SEL in educational contexts. In J. A. Durlak, C. E. Domitrovich, R. P. Weissberg, & T. P. Gullotta (Eds.), *Handbook of social and emotional learning: Research and practice*. The Guilford Press.

Ding, J. (2023, April 26). *How long does it take a business to be profitable? A guide*. FreshBooks. Retrieved January 25, 2024, from https://www.freshbooks.com/hub/startup/how-long-does-it-take-business-to-be-profitable

Durlak, J. A., Weissberg, R. P., Dymnicki, A. B., Taylor, R. D., & Schellinger, K. B. (2011). The impact of enhancing students' social and emotional learning: A meta-analysis of school-based universal interventions. *Child Development, 82*(1), 405–432. https://doi.org/10.1111/j.1467-8624.2010.01564.x

Durlak, J. A., Domitrovich, C. E., Weissberg, R. P., & Gullotta, T. P. (2015). Handbook of social and emotional learning: Research and practice. https://ci.nii.ac.jp/ncid/BB19322885.

Eagle, J. W., Dowd-Eagle, S., Snyder, A., & Holtzman, E. G. (2014). Implementing a multi-tiered system of support (MTSS): Collaboration between school psychologists and administrators to promote systems-level change. *Journal of Educational and Psychological Consultation, 25*(2–3), 160–177. https://doi.org/10.1080/10474412.2014.929960

Freeman, J. L., Sugai, G., Simonsen, B., & Everett, S. (2016). MTSS coaching: Bridging knowing to doing. *Theory Into Practice, 56*(1), 29–37. https://doi.org/10.1080/00405841.2016.1241946

Frieden, T. R. (2014). Six components necessary for effective public health program implementation. *American Journal of Public Health, 104*(1), 17–22. https://doi.org/10.2105/ajph.2013.301608

FSG: Reimagining Social Change. (2016, March 16). *The case for developmental evaluation*. Retrieved September 15, 2024, from https://www.fsg.org/blog/case-developmental-evaluation/

Hunter, D. M., & Mpofu, Z. (2022). Leveraging collective impact to address structural racism in Buncombe County, North Carolina. *Journal of Public Health Management and Practice: JPHMP, 28*(Suppl 1), S38–S42. https://doi.org/10.1097/PHH.0000000000001434

Hunter, W. C., Maheady, L., Jasper, A., Williamson, R. L., Murley, R. C., & Stratton, E. (2015). Numbered heads together as a tier 1 instructional strategy in multitiered systems of support. *Education and Treatment of Children, 38*(3), 345–362. https://doi.org/10.1353/etc.2015.0017

Institute for Healthcare Improvement. (IHI). (2003). *The breakthrough series: IHI's collaborative model for achieving breakthrough improvement.* IHI Innovation Series white paper. Retrieved September 18, 2024, from https://www.ihi.org/resources/white-papers/breakthrough-series-ihis-collaborative-model-achieving-breakthrough

Kania, J., & Kramer, M. (2011, Winter). Collective impact. *Stanford Social Innovation Review*. Retrieved September 18, 2023, from https://ssir.org/articles/entry/collective_impact

Kania, J., Williams, J., Schmitz, P., Brady, S., Kramer, M., & Juster, J. S. (2022, Winter). Centering equity in collective impact. *Stanford Social Innovation Review.* Retrieved February 7, 2024, from https://ssir.org/articles/entry/centering_equity_in_collective_impact

Kessler, R. C., Berglund, P. A., Demler, O. V., Jin, R., Merikangas, K. R., & Walters, E. E. (2005). Lifetime prevalence and age-of-onset distributions of DSM-IV disorders in the National Comorbidity Survey Replication. *Archives of General Psychiatry, 62*(6), 593. https://doi.org/10.1001/archpsyc.62.6.593

Landers, E., Courtade, G. R., & Ryndak, D. L. (2012). Including students with severe disabilities in school-wide positive behavioral interventions and supports: Perceptions of state coordinators. *Research and Practice for Persons with Severe Disabilities, 37*(1), 1–8. https://doi.org/10.2511/027494812800903256

Marmot, M. & Wilkinson, R.G., Editors. (1999). Social determinants of health. .

Massachusetts General Hospital: Psychiatry. (n.d.) *Pediatric symptom checklist.* Retrieved April 12, 2024, from https://www.massgeneral.org/psychiatry/treatments-and-services/pediatric-symptom-checklist

Mellon, E. (2016, December 5). Local nonprofit may have an answer for district's poor exams record. *Houston Chronicle*. https://www.houstonchronicle.com/news/houston-texas/education/article/Local-nonprofit-may-have-an-answer-for-district-s-10691333.php

Mental Health America. (2023). *State of mental health in America*. Youth Ranking 2023. Retrieved May 7, 2024, from https://www.mhanational.org/issues/2023/mental-health-america-youth-data

MTSS (Massachusetts Department of Elementary and Secondary Education (DESE). (2023). *Social, Emotional and Behavioral (SEB) Academy: Needs assessment and planning process*. MA DESE. Retrieved March 29, 2024, from https://www.doe.mass.edu/sfss/mtss/

Musgrove, M. (2011). *A response to intervention (RTI) process cannot be used to delay-deny an evaluation for eligibility under the Individuals with Disabilities Education Act (IDEA)* (11th–07 ed.). United States Department of Education – Office of Special Education and Rehabilitative Services.

National Academies of Sciences, Engineering, and Medicine; Health and Medicine Division; Division of Behavioral and Social Sciences and Education; Board on Children, Youth, and Families; Committee on Applying Lessons of Optimal Adolescent Health to Improve Behavioral Outcomes for Youth, Kahn, N. F., & Graham, R. (Eds.). (2019). *Promoting positive adolescent health behaviors and outcomes: Thriving in the 21st century*. National Academies Press.

National Center for Environmental Health. (2017, April 6). *Picture of America: Prevention*. Centers for Disease Control and Prevention. Retrieved September 9, 2023, from https://www.cdc.gov/pictureofamerica/pdfs/Picture_of_America_Prevention.pdf

Nelson, J. R., Benner, G. J., Lane, K. L., & Smith, B. (2004). Academic achievement of K-12 students with emotional and behavioral disorders. *Exceptional Children, 71*(1), 59–73. https://doi.org/10.1177/001440290407100104

Nobre, J., Oliveira, A. P., Monteiro, F., Sequeira, C., & Ferré-Grau, C. (2021). Promotion of mental health literacy in adolescents: A scoping review. *International Journal of Environmental Research and Public Health, 18*(18), 9500. https://doi.org/10.3390/ijerph18189500

Owens, P. L., Hoagwood, K., Horwitz, S. M., Leaf, P. J., Poduska, J. M., Kellam, S. G., & Ialongo, N. S. (2002). Barriers to children's mental health services. *Journal of the American Academy of Child and Adolescent Psychiatry, 41*(6), 731–738. https://doi.org/10.1097/00004583-200206000-00013

Panorama Education. (n.d.). *Proud partner to Texas districts*. PanoramaED. https://www.panoramaed.com/state/texas?state=texas

PowerSchool. (n.d.). *PowerSchool & kickboard: A more comprehensive approach to understanding and supporting the whole child*. Retrieved April 12, 2024, from https://www.powerschool.com/Kickboard/

Prisco, V., Prisco, L., & Donnarumma, B. (2020). Telepsichiatria negli adulti e negli adolescenti: uno strumento utile contro la CoViD-19 [Telepsychiatry in adults and adolescents: a useful tool against CoViD-19.]. *Recenti Progressi in Medicina, 111*(7), 411–414. https://doi.org/10.1701/3407.33923

Schor, E. L. (2024). Capitated, multisector, universal preventive health care for children and youth. *JAMA Pediatrics*. https://doi.org/10.1001/jamapediatrics.2023.5929

Second Step: Middle School Curriculum. (2024). *CASEL program guide*. Retrieved May 7, 2024, from https://pg.casel.org/second-step-middle-school-curriculum/

Shultz, J. M., Sullivan, L. M., & Galea, S. (2021). *Public health: An introduction to the science and practice of population health*. Springer.

Stiffman, A. R., Stelk, W., Horwitz, S. M., Evans, M. E., Outlaw, F. H., & Atkins, M. (2010). A public health approach to children's mental health services: Possible solutions to current service inadequacies. *Administration and Policy in Mental Health, 37*(1–2), 120–124. https://doi.org/10.1007/s10488-009-0259-2

StriveTogether. (2024). *Theory of action: Pillars "evidence-based decision making" and "collaborative action"; gateways "sustaining" and "systems change"*. Retrieved April 13, 2024, from https://www.strivetogether.org/what-we-do/theory-of-action/

StriveTogether. (n.d.). *StriveTogether: Every child. Cradle to career.* https://www.strivetogether.org/

Sugai, G. (2018). Key questions and detailed answers about PBIS. PBIS.org. Retrieved September 9, 2023, from https://www.gadoe.org/Curriculum-Instruction-and-Assessment/Curriculum-and-Instruction/Documents/New%20Curriculum%20Directors/WhatisPBIS-QandADoc_Sugai2018.pdf

Sugai, G., & Horner, R. (2009). Responsiveness-to-intervention and school-wide positive behavior supports: Integration of multi-tiered system approaches. *Exceptionality, 17*(4), 223–237. https://doi.org/10.1080/09362830903235375

The Fourth R. (2024). *CASEL program guide*. Retrieved May 7, 2024, from https://pg.casel.org/the-fourth-r/

Trafalis, S., Giannini, C., Joves, J., Portera, S., Toyama, H., Mehta, A., Basile, K., & Friedberg, R. D. (2021). A pediatrician-friendly review of three common behavioral health screeners in pediatric practice: Findings and recommendations. *Pediatric Investigation, 5*(1), 58–64. https://doi.org/10.1002/ped4.12246

U.S. Department of Education. (2011, January 21). *MEMO: OSEP memo 11-07 response to intervention (RTI).* Retrieved April 7. 2024, from https://sites.ed.gov/idea/idea-files/osep-memo-11-07-response-to-intervention-rti-memo/

University of Michigan Department of Education. (n.d.). Retrieved April 10, 2023, from https://www.michigan.gov/mde/resources/michigans-top-10-strategic-education-plan/definitions/whole-child.

What is PBIS? (n.d.). *PBIS rewards*. Retrieved September 18, 2023, from https://www.pbisrewards.com/blog/what-is-pbis/

Chapter 7
Global Adolescent Mental Health

Arthur Maerlender and Patricia Gail Bray

7.1 Introduction

The World Health Organization has demonstrated significant leadership in advocating for the implementation of mental health programs worldwide. As early as 1986, the Jakarta Declaration of the World Health Organization (WHO, 2009) emphasized the important role of the settings in which the prerequisites of health are created as critical for implementing effective approaches to health promotion. Schools were identified as the primary setting for health promotion among youth and adolescents. Several international meetings have reiterated this position. The purpose of this chapter is to provide an overview of global adolescent mental health and to highlight recommendations that can be applied in the USA and other countries.

Describing the adolescent mental health crisis and explaining the causes are two different issues. Elements that may seem obvious abound: climate anxiety, erosion of civil discourse, and increase in aggressive acts, social media, and misinformation. However, empirical evidence is difficult to obtain given the worldwide scope. Two scholars in England have added a novel hypothesis to this mix: mental health prevalence inflation (Foulkes & Andrews, 2023). They propose that ironically the increase in adolescent mental health problems may be due in part to the success of efforts to improve the recognition and acceptance of mental health issues. They posited two mechanisms to account for this. One is that accurate reporting and

A. Maerlender (✉)
Department of Psychology, Saint Anselm College, Manchester, NH, USA

Center for Brain, Biology and Behavior, University of Nebraska – Lincoln, Lincoln, NE, USA
e-mail: amaerlender@anselm.edu; amaerlender2@unl.edu

P. G. Bray
Department of Management, Policy and Community Health, UTHealth Houston School of Public Health, The University of Texas Health Science Center (UTHealth) at Houston, Houston, TX, USA

P. G. Bray, A. Maerlender (eds.), *Adolescent Public Mental Health*,
https://doi.org/10.1007/978-3-031-68294-0_7

better recognition are a direct result of global efforts (Wellcome Global Monitor Project, 2020). Improved recognition is a positive factor in its own right, allowing individuals to recognize and report mental health problems previously unreported. While *improved recogni*tion may be driving increases, the authors do not suggest these efforts should be stopped. This phenomenon is well known in other medical domains such as autism (Chiarotti & Venerosi, 2020) and mild traumatic brain injury (concussions) (Bell et al., 2017).

The second mechanism is *overinterpretation*. "This proposes that awareness efforts are leading some individuals to unnecessarily consider milder or more transient psychological difficulties as mental health problems that require labelling, reporting and treating – i.e. problems of living that were not previously considered mental health problems" (Foulkes & Andrews, 2023, p 1). This mechanism was described as more problematic than improved recognition but is a consequence of it because of the potential of individuals to over-pathologize what may be common psychological experiences. By interpreting life difficulties as pathological signs or symptoms, it becomes a self-fulfilling prophecy complete with changes in self-concept and/or behavior that ultimately create or exacerbate symptoms of mental illness.

The authors' final prediction is that the relationship between mental health awareness through improved recognition efforts that sensitizes individuals to a point of worry has served to (inadvertently) increase rates of mental health problems in a cyclical and escalating spiral. The authors are quite clear that this process is speculative and requires validation. Yet it does suggest that a more positive focus on improving well-being may be a needed counterweight to the possible risks of overinterpretation. The shift toward well-being includes providing education and services in schools.

7.2 Mental Health Action Plan

In 2020, the World Health Organization published the *Mental Health Atlas* to address gaps in mental health information (WHO, 2021b). The objectives of this project included collecting, compiling, and disseminating relevant information about mental health resources across the 194 member states. Based on the information gathered by the *Atlas*, the WHO instituted a "Comprehensive Mental Health Action Plan 2013–2020" (WHO, 2021a). The *WHO Mental Health Atlas* has become the best known and is the most extensive source of member state-reported information on mental health resources, aggregated across six WHO regions. The WHO (2021a, p. 5) action plan included the following objectives:

1. To strengthen effective leadership and governance for mental health.
2. To provide comprehensive, integrated, and responsive mental health and social care services in community-based settings.
3. To implement strategies for promotion and prevention in mental health.
4. To strengthen information systems, evidence, and research for mental health.

These objectives have associated global targets in order to measure collective action and achievement by the member states over time. The WHO (2021a, p. 5) action plan outlines six principles and approaches for mental health strategies, actions, and interventions, including the following:

1. Access to universal health coverage.
2. Comply with human rights.
3. Use scientific evidence and/or best practice.
4. Take a life-course approach that recognizes all stages of life.
5. Partner with public and private multisectors.
6. Empower those with mental disorders and psychosocial disabilities.

Globally, efforts with similar themes of mental illness prevention together with proactive supports for well-being are being developed and implemented across the world (WHO, 2021a). According to the *WHO Mental Health Atlas 2020* (WHO, 2021b), 146 countries out of 194 completed reports stating that they have a policy plan for mental health. Of those with a plan, 99 are in compliance with human rights instruments. Fewer than half of those (41) are both fully compliant and engaged in a process of implementation. Of those, only 37 have reported on the use of selected indicators to monitor the implementation efforts (WHO, 2021b). Country-specific details are not presented.

Four-hundred and twenty (420) programs reported to provide mental health promotion and prevention. Of those, 18% were aimed at improving mental health awareness or combating stigma, 17% were school-based mental health prevention and promotion programs, and 15% were aimed at suicide prevention. Slightly more than half of the countries reported having mental health policy plans in place for adolescents (53%). The Southeast Asia region, however, reported that 100% of their responding countries had policy plans in place for adolescents.

In the *Atlas* survey, countries were asked to identify ongoing collaborations between government mental health services at the national level and other ministries, services, and sectors. They were also asked to identify the number and type of stakeholder groups currently collaborating with government mental health services in the planning and/or delivery of mental health promotion, prevention, treatment, and rehabilitation services. Although the numbers dropped between 2017 and 2020 due to the pandemic, 76% of countries reported formal collaborations with at least one stakeholder group (down from 81% in 2017). In regard to specific stakeholders, 42% reported formal collaborations with education ministries or departments. Half of those were functioning mental health prevention and promotion programs, signifying the importance of prevention.

7.2.1 Country-Specific Metrics

Although the *WHO Mental Health Atlas* is a valuable global database, comparable, global mental health data at the country level is sporadic at best, with few exceptions. The Global Mind Project is one of those exceptions.

The Mental State of the World Report is the annual report of the Global Mind Project (Sapien Labs, 2024) and provides trends and insights on the mental well-being of Internet-enabled populations around the globe. In 2023, they collected data from over 500,000 respondents in 13 languages across 71 countries that spanned 9 regions. Global data is collected using the Mental Health Quotient (MHQ) assessment, a comprehensive online survey of cognitive and emotional capabilities that provides an overall mental well-being metric (the MHQ score) as well as multiple dimensional views that relate to the ability to navigate the normal stresses of life and function productively.

The higher the score, the better the mental health of a country, on average. In Table 7.1, four gross national income per capita classifications based on World Bank (2022) data are presented and include (1) lower income countries, (2) lower middle-income countries, (3) upper middle-income countries, and (4) upper income countries. Of the 71 countries with an MHQ score, a sample of 20 countries are represented here. Five countries from each income category are shown as examples.

The revelation is that income only accounts for 5.1% of the variation in the MHQ. In other words, some low-income countries have high scores and some high-income countries have low scores, but it is not a stable inverse relationship. The highest MHQ scores can be found in countries in the lower income categories, including the Dominican Republic, Sri Lanka, and Tanzania (Sapien Labs, 2024). Each has considerably lower gross national income per capita, when compared with any in the highest income category. Although the relationship between poverty and mental health has been studied for the past three decades (Lund et al., 2010), perhaps by examining the particular dimensions of income and poverty, the reasons behind the conundrum illustrated in this table will be illuminated.

7.3 Adolescent Mental Health

Based on the WHO action plan principles, and together with the United Nations International Children's Emergency Fund (UNICEF), the WHO developed a joint program on mental health and psychosocial well-being and development of children and adolescents (WHO, 2022). The objectives included in Box 7.1 mirrors the recommendations identified in the earlier WHO (2021a) action plan.

Box 7.1: WHO and UNICEF Adolescent Mental Health Recommendations (WHO, 2022)

1. Strengthen leadership, governance, and advocacy by developing multisector, multi-stakeholder collaborations.
2. Strengthen service delivery and care systems by improving access to and quality of services.
3. Promotion and prevention in mental health by expanding supportive and nurturing environments.
4. Strengthen information systems, evidence, and research to develop evidence and inform multisector actions and policies.

Table 7.1 Sampling of countries with World Bank 2022 FY gross national income per capita and average Mental Health Quotient

Lower income (≤$1210)			Lower middle income ($2820–$4100)			Upper middle income ($8140–$12,920)			Upper income ($49,240 or more)		
Country	US$	MHQ	Country	US$	MHQ	Country	US$	MHQ	Country	US$	MHQ
Mozambique	440	70	Bangladesh	2820	62	Brazil	8140	53	UK	49,240	49
Congo, DR	610	71	Sri Lanka	3610	89	Dominican Republic	9050	91	Germany	54,030	61
Sudan	760	64	Tunisia	3830	67	Argentina	11,590	71	Israel	55,140	77
Tanzania	1200	88	Philippines	3950	78	Malaysia	11,830	85	Australia	60,840	54
Tajikistan	1210	53	Egypt	4100	55	Costa Rica	12,920	81	USA	76,770	72

In 2021, the WHO released a fact sheet on the mental health of adolescents as a response to COVID-19 noting that "[t]he consequences of failing to address adolescent mental health conditions extend to adulthood, impairing both physical and mental health and limiting opportunities to lead fulfilling lives as adults" (WHO, 2021c).

Recognizing adolescence as a crucial period of development, the report highlights the importance of social and emotional development in the service of well-being. Daily living behaviors of sleep, exercise, effective problem-solving and managing, and positive interpersonal relationships are best served through protective and supportive environments of home, school, and community. Factors such as exposure to adversity, pressure to conform with peers, exploration of identity, sexual violence and bullying, harsh parenting, and severe socioeconomic problems contribute to stress and are known risks to positive mental health (WHO, 2021c).

7.4 Adolescent Mental Health and Schools

Health services, health education, and healthy school environments have long been recommended and available to schoolchildren in Western societies (Green & Kreuter, 1999). More comprehensive programs such as the WHO Health Promoting School program (Parsons et al., 1996) and the US Coordinated School Health program (Allensworth & Kolbe, 1987, Marx and Wooley, 1998) moved toward more broad concepts of health.

The WHO-UNICEF plan recognized schools as essential environments and published "Briefing Note for National Governments: Promoting and Protecting Mental Health in Schools and Learning Environments." This plan put forward five essential pillars (UNICEF, 2022):

1. Create an enabling learning environment for positive mental health and well-being.
2. Guarantee access to early intervention and mental health services and support.
3. Promote teacher well-being.
4. Enhance mental health and psychosocial support (MHPSS) capacity in the education workforce.
5. Ensure meaningful collaboration between the school, family, and community to build a safe and nurturing learning environment.

The briefing offers important considerations for implementing programs with a rationale as to why mental health and social support were important in schools and learning environments. It goes on to highlight eight countries that have developed significant programs, including Kazakhstan, Ecuador, Mozambique, Vietnam, Thailand, Egypt, Iran, and Pakistan. This indicates advancement in some of the poorest countries in the world, such as Mozambique, whose gross national income per capita is $440, compared to the USA, which is $76,770 per capita (World Bank, 2022).

Of interest to this volume, the WHO Comprehensive Mental Health Action Plan (2021a) emphasized increased use of evidence-based interventions and principles of graduated care and holistic approaches that combine mental and physical healthcare. Critically, such integrated and responsive forms of care require training and monitoring of nonspecialized health workers together with sensitive methods to identify people with and at-risk for mental health conditions. However, only 21% of countries offered psychosocial interventions.

7.5 The Adolescent Mental Health Crisis Persists

Although the global pandemic exacerbated the trends, increases in adolescent mental illnesses were being documented prior to the pandemic over the past 30 years (Piao et al., 2022). Globally, 8.8% of children and adolescents have been diagnosed with various mental illnesses, with notable increased rates in anxiety disorders, major depressive disorders, and eating disorders. From 1990 to 2019, the age-standardized rates of DALYs[1] of mental disorders increased from 803.8 per 100,000 (95% CI: 567.7–1104.3 per 100,000) to 833.2 per 100,000 (95% CI: 589.0–1146.1 per 100,000) population.

According to the World Health Organization (WHO, 2022), an estimated one in seven adolescents globally experience a mental health disorder, and suicide remains one of the top causes of death among young people aged 15–19 years. Unaddressed mental health issues during adolescence can have severe and long-lasting consequences. Potential problems include impaired social and interpersonal relationships, academic underachievement, unemployment, violence, and substance abuse. Not addressing mental health issues is also a risk factor for developing later-life chronic mental and physical health problems.

Evidence and gap maps (EGM) are interactive tools that identify existing research findings on a topic and point to areas of research need. One such map identified the effective interventions for both promoting mental health and preventing mental illness in children and adolescents from low- and middle-income countries (Yu et al., 2023). Their findings indicated that the majority of research on mental health and psychosocial support (MHPSS) interventions focused on the treatment of disorders (reactive studies) as opposed to mental health promotion and/or prevention (proactive studies). School-based interventions made up 61% of the research; treatment studies were 59% of the studies, with depression treatment the most frequently studied disorder (40%, $N = 282$), followed by anxiety disorders (32%) and PTSD (18%). Well-being was studied in 21% of the studies (Yu et al., 2023).

A caveat in statistical reporting has been explored and noted by Kieling et al. (2024). Estimating prevalence or DALYs can be misleading when looking at broad

[1] Disability-adjusted life years (DALYs) are a measure of overall disease burden, expressed as the number of years lost due to ill-health, disability, or early death.

categories. They estimated global prevalence and DALYs associated with mental disorders and substance use disorders (SUDs) across four age groups using data from the 2019 Global Burden of Disease (GBD) study. The prevalence of each individual disorder varied by age groups with sex-specific patterns varying by age. The estimated prevalence of mental disorders for those aged 10–14 years was 12.40% (95% UI, 10.62–14.59), while for those aged 15–19 years, it was 13.96% (95% UI, 12.36–15.78). Mental disorders accounted for 31.14 million of 153.59 million DALYs (20.27% of DALYs from all causes). SUDs accounted for 4.30 million DALYs (2.80% of DALYs from all causes). Over the entire life course, 24.85% of all DALYs attributable to mental disorders were recorded before age 25 years. Given these increases, Saunders et al. concluded that "(t)he mental health of youth across the globe is in crisis" (Saunders et al., 2023, p. 3).

7.6 From Mental Illness to Well-Being

Indeed, many past efforts have focused primarily on health and health promotion and not well-being (Konu & Rimpelä, 2002). In response, both Europe and the USA have demonstrated signs of a gradual shift in focus from ill-health to well-being (Kapadia, 2024).

In 2021, the WHO held the tenth Global Conference on Health Promotion that focused on well-being, marking the first time that WHO has used well-being as the theme of a major conference. Well-being encompasses quality of life, as well as the ability of people and societies to contribute to the world in accordance with a sense of meaning and purpose. Both physical health and mental health have psychological (inner, subjective) components and social-cultural-environmental (outer, objective) components (WHO, 2021d).

This shift directs attention to a more positive behavioral and psychological direction of change, from curing to prevention, from eliminating a negative state to attaining a positive state. A focus on well-being helps to reduce stigma while promoting an acknowledged benefit to individuals (Carstensen et al., 2011; Chida & Steptoe, 2008) and societies (Livingston et al., 2022).

Key principles for putting effective mental healthcare in place follow public health models. Recommendations on youth mental healthcare place a high priority on mental health promotion as a key prevention tool, while cross-sectional organization and funding of care services are critical components. These include increased flexibility of care settings, early intervention, and a strengths orientation instead of focusing on deficits and diagnoses (Zechmeister-Koss et al., 2023).

The European Commission has specifically shown concern for the well-being of students in European schools:

> A general consensus exists among Member States that gaining academic knowledge on its own is not enough for young people to play a role as active citizens and face the socio-economic realities in their lives, in order to avoid inequity, poverty, discrimination, marginalisation and exclusion. In the 21st century, education needs to go beyond narrow sectoral

> goals such as academic achievement. In addition, it should contribute actively to the health and well-being of children and young people, whose mental health needs are becoming more evident and demanding. (Cefai et al., 2021, p. 10)

Based on their review of the evidence, the European Commission has supported whole-school approach to mental health and well-being (Cefai et al., 2022). A priority is to develop school curriculum that teaches and supports mental health and well-being. Social and emotional education, resilience building, and mental health literacy (including addressing stigma and prejudice) should be developed and adapted to the context and needs of the school. Key to this effort are the following principles:

- Feeling safe, valued, and respected
- Being actively and meaningfully engaged in academic and social activities
- Having positive self-esteem, self-efficacy, and a sense of autonomy
- Having positive and supportive relationships with teachers and peers
- Feeling a sense of belonging to their classroom and school
- Feeling happy and satisfied with their lives at school

In the USA, addressing adolescent mental health through school-based programs, policies, and initiatives has been a key priority, reflecting the pivotal role that educational settings play in the lives of young people (Richter et al., 2022; Rones & Hoagwood, 2000; U.S. Surgeon General, 2021).

While the key principles are slightly different, both the USA and Europe have identified overlapping characteristics for supporting both students and staff in proactive behaviors to enhance health and well-being. The overarching constructs are safety, engagement, self-efficacy, positive relationships, and satisfaction with learning.

Although the USA system is decentralized and not government directed as in many other countries, certain characteristics, including school-based mental health services, seem to be consistent with WHO and European initiatives. Others include integrated care models, wraparound services, and peer support programs. One exception is that the WHO's action plan ranks universal healthcare as the top recommendation, and the USA does not include universal healthcare as a recommendation.

7.7 USA Exemplars

In the USA, addressing adolescent mental health through school-based programs, policies, and initiatives has been a key priority, reflecting the pivotal role that educational settings play in the lives of young people.

To support these changes, the ongoing development of health service professions in the USA and European schools has driven the expanding understanding of the critical role of mental health in the development of children and youth. Together with the realization of the relationships between mental health, physical health, and the social determinants of health, a picture has emerged that highlights the communal matrix of supports needed for optimal well-being along with an awareness of the immense value of educational institutions in that matrix.

Some notable programs in the USA include the National Child Traumatic Stress Network (n.d.), established in 2000 through a congressional initiative, which is a collaboration of academic and community partners that has developed and disseminated evidence-based interventions, resources, and training to support schools in addressing the impact of trauma on students' mental health and learning.

Another initiative, the Project AWARE program (Advancing Wellness and Resilience in Education), funded by the Substance Abuse and Mental Health Services Administration (SAMHSA), provides grants to increase awareness of mental health issues among school-aged youth. Project AWARE promotes the implementation of multitiered system of supports (MTSS). There is also good evidence for programs such as whole-school positive behavioral interventions and supports (PBIS) (Lee & Gage, 2020) and social-emotional learning (SEL) curricula, within school districts and communities (Cipriano et al., 2023).[2]

7.8 USA Mental Health Policy

At the policy level, the USA has made strides in addressing adolescent mental health through legislation such as the Mental Health Reform Act of 2022. This bipartisan bill aims to strengthen the mental health care system, including provisions to support school-based mental health services, expand the mental health workforce, and increase access to telehealth and digital mental health tools.

Furthermore, the Consolidated Appropriations Act of 2023 included significant investments in mental health programs and services for children and youth, including funding for the National Child Traumatic Stress Network, Project AWARE, and youth suicide prevention initiatives.

These various USA initiatives and policy efforts reflect a growing recognition of the importance of addressing adolescent mental health through coordinated, multicomponent strategies that involve schools, healthcare systems, communities, and policymakers. By fostering collaboration across sectors and leveraging the unique role of educational settings, these approaches aim to create a comprehensive system of support that promotes mental wellness, identifies concerns early, and provides appropriate interventions for young people across the continuum of need.

Additionally, from a public health perspective, including indicators of well-being and optimal functioning creates a proactive outcome that is not just the elimination of disease. Preventing illness through education and support for well-being also

---

[2] Social-emotional learning is an educational program like math or reading in which the subject matter is learning to understand and manage emotions, develop positive relationships, be responsible, set goals, and exhibit empathy. A large body of research supports its effectiveness (Greenberg, 2023).

seems less likely to marginalize or stigmatize individuals while addressing core societal challenges posed by the social determinants of health. Schools are where adolescents spend significant time in the activities of learning. And learning how to optimize one's potential, to become resilient, and to nurture one's well-being is an appropriate school function that enhances academic learning.

7.9 Conclusion

Globally, population mental health has been raised as an important concern, with adolescence acknowledged as a critical period for prevention, promotion, and development of positive mental health behaviors and attitudes. Although mental illness had been increasing prior to the pandemic, the worldwide COVID public health crisis exacerbated the incidence rates of problems such as anxiety, depression, suicide, risk taking, and substance abuse. Adolescent mental health is now fully recognized worldwide, and countries are implementing programs to address mental health issues, where, in some places, the mere idea of mental illness has been culturally eschewed.

A shift of focus to both individual and population well-being has been supported by research and is gaining traction. Emerging themes include awareness raising, counselor training, peer education, and integrating services into schools and communities to reach youth. However, lack of resources remains a major challenge for sustained, comprehensive mental health programming in many countries forcing prevention and enhanced well-being to the side for now.

Still, the evidence seems clear that, for adolescents, supportive and nurturing school-based educational programming is important. That programming should address conflict resolution, affect management, relationship building, and goal setting for enhancing positive cognitive, behavioral, and emotional outcomes.

Competing Interests *The authors have no conflicts of interest to declare that are relevant to the content of this chapter.*

References

Allensworth, D. D., & Kolbe, L. J. (1987). The comprehensive school health program: Exploring an expanded concept. *Journal of School Health, 57*(10), 409–412.

Bell, J. M., Breiding, M. J., & DePadilla, L. (2017). CDC's efforts to improve traumatic brain injury surveillance. *Journal of Safety Research, 62*, 253–256. https://doi.org/10.1016/j.jsr.2017.04.002

Carstensen, L. L., Turan, B., Scheibe, S., Ram, N., Ersner-Hershfield, H., Samanez-Larkin, G. R., Brooks, K. P., & Nesselroade, J. R. (2011). Emotional experience improves with age: Evidence based on over 10 years of experience sampling. *Psychology and Aging, 26*(1), 21–33. https://doi.org/10.1037/a0021285

Cefai, C., Simões, C., & Caravita, S. (2021). *A systemic, whole-school approach to mental health and wellbeing in schools in the EU*. NESET report. Publications Office of the European Union.

Cefai, C., Camilleri, L., Bartolo, P., Grazzani, I., Cavioni, V., Conte, E., Ornaghi, V., Agliati, A., Gandellini, S., Tatalovic Vorkapic, S., Poulou, M., Martinsone, B., Stokenberga, I., Simões, C., Santos, M., & Colomeischi, A. A. (2022). The effectiveness of a school-based, universal mental health programme in six European countries. *Frontiers in Psychology, 13*, 925614. https://doi.org/10.3389/fpsyg.2022.925614

Chiarotti, F., & Venerosi, A. (2020). Epidemiology of autism spectrum disorders: A review of worldwide prevalence estimates since 2014. *Brain Sciences, 10*(5), 274. https://doi.org/10.3390/brainsci10050274

Chida, Y., & Steptoe, A. (2008). Positive psychological well-being and mortality: A quantitative review of prospective observational studies. *Psychosomatic Medicine, 70*(7), 741–756. https://doi.org/10.1097/PSY.0b013e31818105ba

Cipriano, C., Strambler, M. J., Naples, L. H., Ha, C., Kirk, M., Wood, M., Sehgal, K., Zieher, A. K., Eveleigh, A., McCarthy, M., Funaro, M., Ponnock, A., Chow, J. C., & Durlak, J. (2023). The state of evidence for social and emotional learning: A contemporary meta-analysis of universal school-based SEL interventions. *Child Development, 94*, 1181–1204. https://doi.org/10.1111/cdev.13968

Foulkes, J. L., & Andrews, J. (2023). Are mental health awareness efforts contributing to the rise in reported mental health problems? A call to test the prevalence inflation hypothesis. *New Ideas in Psychology, 69*, 1–6. https://doi.org/10.1016/j.newideapsych.2023.101010

Green, L. D., & Kreuter, M. W. (1999). *Health promotion planning: An educational and ecological approach* (3rd ed.). Mayfield.

Greenberg, M. T. (2023). Evidence for social and emotional learning in schools. *Learning Policy Institute., 10*(54300/928), 269.

Kapadia, F. (2024). Adolescent mental health and well-being: A public health of consequence. *American Journal of Public Health, 114*(2), 158–160. https://doi.org/10.2105/AJPH.2023.307543

Kieling, C., Buchweitz, C., Caye, A., et al. (2024). Worldwide prevalence and disability from mental disorders across childhood and adolescence: Evidence from the Global Burden of Disease Study. *JAMA Psychiatry*. Advance online publication. https://doi.org/10.1001/jamapsychiatry.2023.5051.

Konu, A., & Rimpelä, M. (2002). Well-being in schools: A conceptual model. *Health Promotion International, 17*(1), 79–87. https://doi.org/10.1093/heapro/17.1.79

Lee, A., & Gage, N. (2020). Updating and expanding systematic reviews and meta-analyses on the effects of school-wide positive behavior interventions and supports. *Psychology in the Schools, 57*. https://doi.org/10.1002/pits.22336

Livingston, V., Jackson-Nevels, B., & Reddy, V. V. (2022). Social, cultural, and economic determinants of well-being. *Encyclopedia, 2*, 1183–1199. https://doi.org/10.3390/encyclopedia2030079

Lund, C., Breen, A., Flisher, A. J., Kakuma, R., Corrigall, J., Joska, J. A., Swartz, L., & Patel, V. (2010). Poverty and common mental disorders in low and middle income countries: A systematic review. *Social Science & Medicine (1982), 71*(3), 517–528. https://doi.org/10.1016/j.socscimed.2010.04.027

Marx, E., & Wooley, S. F. (Eds.). (1998). *Health is academic: A guide to coordinated school health programs*. Teachers College Press.

Parsons, C., Stears, D., & Thomas, C. (1996). The health promoting school in Europe: Conceptualizing and evaluating the change. *Health Education Journal, 55*, 311–321.

Piao, J., Huang, Y., Han, C., et al. (2022). Alarming changes in the global burden of mental disorders in children and adolescents from 1990 to 2019: A systematic analysis for the Global Burden of Disease study. *European Child & Adolescent Psychiatry, 31*(12), 1827–1845. https://doi.org/10.1007/s00787-022-02040-4

Richter, A., Sjunnestrand, M., Romare Strandh, M., & Hasson, H. (2022). Implementing school-based mental health services: A scoping review of the literature summarizing the factors that

affect implementation. *International Journal of Environmental Research and Public Health, 19*(6), 3489. https://doi.org/10.3390/ijerph19063489
Rones, M., & Hoagwood, K. (2000). School-based mental health services: A research review. *Clinical Child and Family Psychology Review, 3*(4), 223–241. https://doi.org/10.1023/A:1026425104386
Sapien Labs. (2024, March 4). *The mental state of the world in 2023: A perspective on internet-enabled populations*. Global Mind Project. Retrieved May 13, 2024, from https://sapienlabs.org/wp-content/uploads/2024/03/4th-Annual-Mental-State-of-the-World-Report.pdf
Saunders, K.R.K., McGuinness, E., Barnett, P., et al. (2023). A scoping review of trauma informed approaches in acute, crisis, emergency, and residential mental health care. *BMC Psychiatry, (23)567*. Retrieved, May 2, 2024, from https://bmcpsychiatry.biomedcentral.com/articles/10.1186/s12888-023-05016-z
The National Child Traumatic Stress Network (NCTSN). (n.d.). Retrieved May 2, 2024, from https://www.nctsn.org/
The Project AWARE (Advancing Wellness and Resiliency in Education). (2022). SAMHSA. Substance Abuse and Mental Health Services Administration. Retrieved May 2, 2024, from https://www.samhsa.gov/grants/grant-announcements/sm-22-001
The World Bank. (2022). *GNI per capita, Atlas method (current US$)—World bank open data: Free and open access to global development data*. Retrieved May 18, 2024, from https://data.worldbank.org/indicator/NY.GNP.PCAP.CD?locations=UG
U.S. Surgeon General. (2021). *Protecting youth mental health: The U.S. Surgeon General's Advisory*. https://www.hhs.gov/sites/default/files/surgeon-general-youth-mental-health-advisory.pdf?null
UNICEF. (United Nations International Children's Fund). (2022). *Five essential pillars for promoting and protecting mental health and psychosocial well-being in schools and learning environments: A briefing for national governments*. Retrieved May 2, 2024, from https://www.unicef.org/media/126821/file/Promoting%20and%20protecting%20mental%20health%20in%20schools%20and%20learning%20environments.pdf
Wellcome Global Monitor Project. (2020). *The role of science in mental health*. Insights from the Wellcome Global Monitor.
WHO. (2009). *Milestones in health promotion statements from global conferences*. World Health Organization. Retrieved April 17, 2024, from https://www.who.int/publications/i/item/WHO-NMH-CHP-09.01
WHO. (2021a). *Comprehensive mental health action plan 2013–2030*. World Health Organization. Licence: CC BY-NC-SA 3.0 IGO. https://iris.who.int/bitstream/handle/10665/345301/9789240031029-eng.pdf?sequence=1
WHO. (2021b). *Mental health atlas 2020*. World Health Organization. Retrieved April 17, 2024, from https://www.who.int/publications/i/item/9789240036703
WHO. (2021c). Mental health of adolescents. 17 November. World Health Organization. Retrieved 17 April 2024, from https://www.who.int/news-room/fact-sheets/detail/adolescent-mental-health
WHO. (2021d). *Health promotion glossary of terms 2021*. World Health Organization. https://www.who.int/publications/i/item/9789240038349. Retrieved 15 April 2024
WHO. (2022). *UNICEF and WHO joint programme on mental health and psychosocial well-being and development of children and adolescents*. Global case for support. Retrieved May 10, 2024, from https://www.who.int/publications/i/item/978924006176
Yu, R., Perera, C., Sharma, M., Ipince, A., Bakrania, S., Shokraneh, F., Sepulveda, J. S. M., & Anthony, D. (2023). Child and adolescent mental health and psychosocial support interventions: An evidence and gap map of low- and middle-income countries. *Campbell Systematic Reviews, 19*(3), e1349. https://doi.org/10.1002/cl2.1349. PMID: 37621301; PMCID: PMC10445093.
Zechmeister-Koss, I., Jeindl, R., & Hofer, V. (2023). Child and adolescent mental health care models: A scoping review. *International Journal of Technology Assessment in Health Care, 39*(S1), S9–S9. https://doi.org/10.1017/S0266462323000727

Chapter 8
Lessons, Part I: Lessons, Limitations, and Funding of the BridgeUp Model

Patricia Gail Bray

8.1 Introduction

The purpose and passion for this book are to share the successes and inspire others with the experiences learned from The Menninger Clinic's innovative BridgeUp Center. The goal is to offer a way forward for how to begin the arduous task of thinking, talking, and acting about how best to connect the oftentimes invisible adolescent emotional, mental, and social world with the visible physical one. A public health approach places emphasis "upstream" from the clinical setting by making prevention vital to health as treatment. Now is the time for changes, according to the American Academy of Pediatrics' (AAP, 2021) adolescent mental health declaration, which supports the thesis that we are on the cusp of a pediatric paradigm shift. Can a seamless approach like the one envisioned by the Institute of Medicine in 1994 be designed and implemented now (Institute of Medicine, 1994)? The BridgeUp case study in an earlier chapter provided a possible road map, with specific public health concepts to successfully operationalize an approach that integrates health promotion, prevention, treatment, and recovery.

Early preventative measures could be implemented instead of taking action when a crisis occurs. Long waits for diagnoses lead to more severe cases with longer recoveries. Still, there are many structural, cultural, and professional barriers that stand in the way. One early suggestion was to align preventive interventions according to child and adolescent development phases, as recommended by the National Research Council (O'Connell et al., 2009). Another suggestion could include a

P. G. Bray (✉)
Department of Management, Policy and Community Health, UTHealth Houston School of Public Health, The University of Texas Health Science Center (UTHealth) at Houston, Houston, TX, USA
e-mail: Patricia.G.Bray@uth.tmc.edu

P. G. Bray, A. Maerlender (eds.), *Adolescent Public Mental Health*,
https://doi.org/10.1007/978-3-031-68294-0_8

preliminary mental health screen as part of an annual well-child exam, similar to vision and hearing screens.

This chapter summarizes the lessons learned during the 7-year demonstration project at the BridgeUp Center at The Menninger Clinic (BridgeUp) (The first year of the project focused on planning the intervention, funding and evaluation components). The lessons include aspects of the program that needed improvement and aspects that worked well with the intervention. The BridgeUp model, described in a previous chapter, forms the basis for the proposed, new adolescent public mental health (APMH) model. Additional focus is on limitations and funding. Implementation of the BridgeUp model consisted of two phases, each lasting for 3 years. The first phase was the Pilot Phase (Phase I), including the academic years from 2016 to 2019. The second phase was the Strategic, Sustainability, and Scalability Phase (Phase II), including the academic years from 2019 to 2022. The basic structure of the BridgeUp model remained the same for both phases. There were three evidence-based frameworks: integrated social and emotional learning (SEL), multitiered system of supports (MTSS), and multisector collaboration using collective impact (CI). The BridgeUp model was designed to work at the intersection of the three, core systems: adolescent mental health, public health, and school health.[1]

As detailed in an earlier chapter, integrating three large systems at the intersection of adolescent mental health is a more fundamental challenge. The good news is that the frameworks worked well together. The school health chapter earlier in this volume speaks about the benefits of integrating SEL and MTSS. BridgeUp took that idea one step further by expanding the frameworks to include a public health approach, which highlights prevention and the social determinants of health (SDOH).

8.1.1 Background

BridgeUp began at The Menninger Clinic in 2015. The goals were to create a new model using an innovative approach to move upstream from the hospital and focus on adolescent mental health prevention and early intervention in underserved communities. Based on the research, 50% of mental illnesses are diagnosed by age 14 (Kessler et al., 2005), so why not find ways to prevent, screen, and identify early mental health challenges among adolescents? Additionally, the intent was to implement this new model in low-income, disadvantaged areas where most families did not have access to health or mental health services.

After intensive research, the BridgeUp leadership team developed a model drawn from three evidence-based frameworks:

1. Social and emotional learning (SEL). Just a few months after BridgeUp began, dramatic changes occurred at the federal level when the *No Child Left Behind Act* (NCLB) (2001) was replaced by the *Every Student Succeeds Act* (ESSA) (U.S. Department of Education, 2015). ESSA required measuring noncognitive

[1] Note that the concepts, frameworks, and systems are discussed in earlier chapters in this volume.

student skills, thus opening doors to social and emotional learning (SEL). The BridgeUp team chose the Collaborative for Academic and Social and Emotional Learning (CASEL) SEL platform, based on the long history of research and implementation for social and emotional education (Durlak et al., 2015). The CASEL conceptual and competency developments were evidence-based and replicable. That worked for the first tier of the BridgeUp model, since the SEL curriculum addressed skills that enhanced mental health literacy.

2. Multitiered system of supports (MTSS) is a public health approach to improve student outcomes in schools. Aimed for the whole child, the BridgeUp model integrated SEL with MTSS. The MTSS framework worked well for all BridgeUp partners, and a few schools already had the framework in place, as follows in Box 8.1.

3. Collective impact (CI). Multisector collaboration was the third framework for the BridgeUp model. The BridgeUp team chose the CI framework developed by Kania and Kramer (2011). A mental health provider was required as one of the partners for each school-based program.
   CI requires five steps to have a successful, complex systems-change project (Kania & Kramer, 2011). Box 8.2 contains a summary of the collective impact characteristics.

Box 8.1: The BridgeUp MTSS Framework

Primary prevention	Tier 1	SEL instruction to enhance mental health literacy for the whole class or school
Secondary prevention	Tier 2	Small group interventions for students who need additional mental health supports
Tertiary prevention	Tier 3	Intensive individualized support, including mental health referrals for assessment and/or treatment. BridgeUp required the grantees to partner with a mental health provider

Box 8.2: Collective Impact Characteristics

1. All participants have a common agenda for change including a shared understanding of the problem and a joint approach to solving it through agreed upon actions.
2. Collecting data and measuring results consistently across all the participants and ensuring a shared measurement system for alignment and accountability.
3. A plan of action that outlines and coordinates mutually reinforcing activities for each participant.
4. Open and continuous communication is needed across the many players to build trust, assure mutual objectives, and create common motivation.
5. A backbone organization with staff and specific set of skills to serve the entire initiative and coordinate participating organizations and agencies.

Source: Kania and Kramer (2011)

Integrating three frameworks to form a new model is ambitious and fraught with potential risks and limitations (McGill et al., 2021). As with all demonstration projects, there were challenges, lessons learned, limitations, and funding concerns, as reported in this chapter.

8.2 Lessons Learned from the BridgeUp Demonstration Project

Phase I began with development of an extensive Request for Proposal (RFP) process, which continued to be revised during the first 3 years. The revisions were based on lessons learned each year from the multisector partnerships that were funded annually. The partnerships consisted of schools, nonprofits, and mental health providers. Phase II began in the fall semester of 2019, with COVID-19 occurring during the spring of 2020. The RFP requirements remained stable throughout the duration of the project. Addressing the extraordinary mental health, public health, and school health challenges due to COVID-19 served as a good test for the model's resiliency. The lessons learned during Phase II took a different form, focused not so much on the partnership organizations but rather on the emotional and mental well-being of the teachers, administrators, students, and their families.

The lessons learned throughout the implementation were documented in various forms, including a robust, mixed method evaluation plan and established communication paths via regular convenings.[2] The evaluation plan included two levels of measurement: (1) project implementation in the schools by the partnerships, and (2) the BridgeUp Center. The first level consisted of a quantitative and qualitative midyear and annual evaluation report for each of the partnerships. A rapid cycle improvement (RCI) evaluation was added for each partnership during the second year and remained throughout the life of the project. On average, the RCI was completed and reviewed on a monthly basis by each partnership.

The second level of the evaluation included operational metrics and the aggregate program evaluation from the partnerships. These data served to demonstrate the BridgeUp Center's accountability and transparency throughout the project. With both of these approaches, outcomes could be assessed to determine necessary interim corrections. The discussion will highlight where each level needed improvement and what worked well.

In total, there were 46 BridgeUp funded and completed interventions that were implemented in 160 schools over a 6-year period.

[2] The evaluation plan is detailed in an earlier chapter.

8.2.1 What Needed Improvement for the Partnerships: School and School District Considerations

Working in low-income areas, under-resourced schools required respect for diversity and equity concerns. Therefore, the size, culture, demographics, and geographic location of the school/district must be considered when choosing SEL curricula and partners. Additional resources must be included for under-resourced and low-performing schools.

It is strongly recommended that schools be the fiscal agent of the funding. Otherwise, funding to nonprofit organizations that provide programming in schools lacks the authority to require schools to support and sustain the programming.

Multiple interventions were provided to schools that were rated as "Improvement Required" by the Texas Department of Education. These were schools that had not passed state testing requirements for multiple years and were under significant scrutiny to improve test scores. During Phase I, one of the partners reported extensive operational challenges with the school. The partner had to modify the BridgeUp implementation plan in an "Improvement Required" school because there were so many restrictions, such as those related to intervention programs. In another school, both teachers and students experienced difficulty managing behavior; turnover was high for both teachers and adminstrators, creating an unstable environment for the students. The grant partners adapted the program to include a mindful practice at the beginning of the SEL sessions. Improvements were observed, and the partners developed stronger relationships with the principal and school district.

During Phase I, several partners reported difficulty working in multiple schools. Not all sites progressed at the same time, especially regarding program buy-in, support, and implementation. Several sites reported limited programming time due to school or after-school schedules. Some sites have programming only 1 day a week. However, it was not effective to deliver a comprehensive SEL program in one session per week. Partners worked with school administrators to identify additional time for programming. In this context, the same SEL curriculum should be used within school districts for all secondary schools.

Not all partners agreed on solutions to unplanned conflicts that would arise, such as disagreements between the primary intervention partner and the mental literacy partner. One of the BridgeUp leadership team members was a trained mediator and led a series of meetings to resolve thorny disagreements. The requirements of the project must plan for contingencies and unplanned interruptions, such as hurricanes or a global pandemic.

8.2.2 *What Worked Well for the Partnerships: SEL*

This new model required integration across the three different frameworks, so implementation of the BridgeUp model required increased attention from the schools and nonprofits. The Request for Proposal (RFP) was rigorous, and the schools and nonprofits that applied were intrepid. The success of this demonstration project is due to their interest and efforts. This was especially true for the inaugural year.

Grant partners provided SEL programs and activities for all students in their selected schools. The RFP requirements included classroom-based programming using evidence-informed curricula and instruction that aligned with CASEL. Training and coaching for administrators, teachers, and other school- and campus-based personnel were provided to build SEL competence and capacity to teach and model SEL. The SEL skills enhanced mental health literacy and served as a Tier 1 prevention for students. As noted earlier, when *Every Student Succeeds Act* (ESSA) legislation was passed in December 2015, schools were required to include "noncognitive" content into the curriculum. The new noncognitive requirements opened the door for schools to teach students about social and emotional concepts. Not only did this help to bolster students' ability to enjoy healthier relationships informed with better decision-making skills, but the timing was serendipitous for implementation of the BridgeUp model.

SEL served as the basis for mental health literacy in the schools. After the first 2 years, all students received SEL program instruction. The BridgeUp model augmented SEL with MTSS. The following are the highlights from the implementation of SEL as the preventative component.

1. After the inaugural year, all SEL programs were required to choose a Collaborative for Academic and Social and Emotional Learning (CASEL) evidence-informed or evidence-based curriculum. As new research was published, the BridgeUp RFP was modified to account for the evolving best practices.
2. In the first year of the implementation, most of the SEL programs were implemented in after-school programs, and this changed for the remainder of the project to a whole-school approach. Based on new research, during Phase II, a whole-district approach was recommended and preferred.
3. During Phase II, BridgeUp provided capacity building to train teachers and staff about SEL concepts, since this explicit instructional format was not originally part of their college training and credentials. All grants conducted SEL training for teachers and administrators over the summer or early in the school year. The trainings were welcomed and valued, serving 670 adults during the first year. One teacher reported, "My partnership with the SEL program has impacted my teaching by making me more self-aware of my daily interactions with students and strengthening my relationship with them. I have become very intentional about how I communicate expectations and express belief statements in a genu-

ine manner. I also have become comfortable with demonstrating vulnerability and modeling how vulnerability is a sign of inner strength" (BridgeUp at Menninger, 2016–2022).

4. Many schools typically launch initiatives aimed at promoting student achievement and well-being. A key aspect of integrating SEL into the classroom-based curricula created an opportunity for students to engage in open discussions that included emotional and social challenges. Literature is a great entree to these types of guided discussions. For example, one of the most assigned readings in middle school is the Pulitzer Prize winning book, *To Kill a Mockingbird* (1960). A common theme throughout this book is that the widowed father teaches his two young children about empathy and justice. Empathy is included as part of the competencies in the CASEL-5 Wheel. These kinds of examples can be woven into all classes, including science, social studies, and art. An example is included in Box 8.3.
5. Another benefit to SEL instruction interwoven throughout the school day is that children have access to adults trained in SEL. These program leaders and/or teachers can observe students in a safe environment to discern if any children need mental health supports. And the student has an opportunity to be connected to other adults in the school.
6. Other benefits included better attendance and behavior and improved class engagement. Students looked forward to BridgeUp programs as shown by high attendance rates and class engagement in the first year of implementation. For example, one charter middle school reported 98% attendance rate for class sessions and 90% for after-school programming (BridgeUp at Menninger, 2016–2022).

Box 8.3: Example of SEL Instruction in Science Class

One significant grantee partnership was with a local theater organization. They implemented the BridgeUp model at a low-performing, inner-city school in Houston Independent School District. This school had a high turnover rate for administrators and teachers. These students learned about SEL during science class by using dramatic arts to demonstrate various CASEL-5 competencies, which included self-awareness, self-management, social-awareness, how to have healthy relationships, and responsible decision-making. For example, the program director would have students act out the relationship of the planets within the solar system while teaching them about astronomy, and they also learned concepts applicable to the importance of social awareness. The students were engaged and communicative, with improved outcomes, such as attendance.

8.2.3 What Needed Improvement for the Partnerships and MTSS

1. Partners struggled with developing a theory of change model, creating an organizational Logic Model and Rapid Cycle Improvement metrics. The Impact Network consisted of quarterly convenings of the partners. These sessions were instrumental in instructing the partners about how best to improve the implementation with shared decision-making and more relevant metrics.
2. Based on the total number of students during the final year of the project, 2021–2022, the expected number of students referred for mental health supports was lower. With a total of 18,594 students, the expectation was that the total number of students needing additional mental supports ranged from 1116 to 2789. Only 1427 Tiers 2 and 3 students were referred for additional mental health supports, which is much lower than expected. While this represents almost 8% for the entire cohort, there is wide variation in the percentage of referrals. For example, a large school district reported 33% referrals for Tiers 2 and 3, while a medium-sized school district reported only 3%. This is a concern that needs to be addressed in the future. The national average is between 15% and 20%. The referral protocols may need to be standardized across the schools.

8.2.4 What Worked Well for the Partnerships: Mental Health Providers

The funding plan was originally designed to invest more resources in Phase I so that there would be a larger, diverse set of partners to learn about the strengths and weaknesses of the BridgeUp model early on. The success of the project was due, in part, to consistent partners, such as contracting with the same mental health providers each year. The model worked well in Phase II with small, incremental adjustments, despite COVID-19.

1. From the beginning of Phase I, the Request for Proposal (RFP) required mental health providers to become partners on the BridgeUp grant. The leadership anticipated few schools and nonprofits would be able to accommodate this request, but this turned out as predicted, with no challenges recruiting interested mental health providers.
2. The BridgeUp model required the integration of a formal "multitiered system of supports" (MTSS) as part of secondary prevention with SEL. The referrals worked well because of the number of adults working with the students for the SEL component. All BridgeUp schools developed culturally appropriate mental health referral protocols, which provided a process for identifying, referring, and assessing kids who needed additional help. To help align MTSS with the local school programs, a plethora of approaches existed, including positive behavioral

interventions and supports (PBIS), restorative practices, service learning, mindfulness, mentoring, and behavioral health programs.

3. The national average of the percentage of students typically served in Tier 2 is approximately 5–10% of the cohort (CASEL, 2019). Before COVID-19, the BridgeUp prevalence percentages aligned closely with the national norm. After COVID-19, the pattern of disruption showed inconsistency in the number of students referred for mental health supports. This was due to students not attending school during 2020 because of COVID-19. And since 2021 was more of a hybrid year, there was more variation in the data on all levels.
4. Of the 63,325 students participating in the BridgeUp program from 2015 to 2022, 6232 or about 10% of the students were referred to either Tier 2 or Tier 3 for additional mental health supports, reflecting a lower response than the national average. These underserved adolescents typically did not have health insurance or health access to mental health providers. The fact that so many students were provided care is one of the most successful outcomes of the BridgeUp project and exceeded the leadership team's expectations.
5. The BridgeUp model required grantee partners to develop a Tier 3 referral protocol for mental health services for students who did not respond to either Tier 1 primary or Tier 2 secondary prevention, interventions, and supports. Students who needed more intensive mental health supports, such as a formal assessment, therapy, or inpatient care, were referred to community mental health partners or to The Menninger Clinic. These Tier 3 students typically represent 1–5% of those served (CASEL, 2019). The overall number of BridgeUp Tier 3 students averaged 4%.
6. Students living in disadvantaged or underserved communities did not have private insurance or the means to pay for mental health treatment. BridgeUp referred 110 of those who needed intensive supports to Menninger for treatment. The costs were covered partially through pre-allocated BridgeUp funding. Those families who qualified for financial assistance were eligible to receive treatment at no cost, paid for through the federally mandated charity care allocations. Barriers to care, such as transportation issues, stigma, scheduling limitations, or fear, meant that approximately 70% of those referred did not follow through with appointments at Menninger. This is lower than the national average, which is worthy of more research.
7. Barriers that face adolescents seeking mental healthcare and services are covered in a later chapter.
8. Maintaining strong communication pathways is necessary for the duration of the project, so that when needed in times of emergencies, those relationships can work together to address the needs of the students. For example, when COVID-19 happened and the schools closed, a BridgeUp scenario planning team was convened to plan seven different scenarios for how to keep the BridgeUp project going (Neiner et al., 2004).
9. A best practice now, as noted by Simonsen et al. (2021), is that an MTSS framework in schools should be a part of the "implementation cascade," including the classroom, school, district, and state. During Phase II, the BridgeUp model was

implemented in classrooms, whole schools, and, in a few cases, district-wide. There was a formal goal to scale the BridgeUp model statewide, but due to COVID-19, that was not possible.

8.2.5 What Worked Well for the BridgeUp Center: Collective Impact

As part of the BridgeUp model, a CI approach was required. The grant leads obtained signed MOUs before the beginning of the academic year with all partners, including the mental health providers. The grants that worked the best had more than one mental health partner, including private and public entities.

A common agenda is what holds the collaboration together. The agenda was clearly articulated through an RFP process that stipulated how the BridgeUp model was to be used, and yet didn't dictate to the collaboratives how specific procedures would be implemented. This allowed for adaptations based on school diversity, culture, size, and geographic location.

Due to the wide variation in schools and school districts, their measurement systems continued to be developed independently of BridgeUp. However, there were common metrics required for all of the collaboratives. This allowed for midcourse corrections and helped to measure the overall impact of the systems change.

BridgeUp served as the backbone support for the design, development, funding, implementation, and evaluation for the BridgeUp project. The program implementation represented multisector collaboratives, which included schools, nonprofit organizations, and mental health providers. The backbone role was important on two levels: 1) BridgeUp convened the partners together regularly throughout the academic year which created and reinforced opportunities for shared learnings and innovations, and 2) BridgeUp served as a problem-solver and mediator when conflicts arose.

As an extension of the CI approach, the BridgeUp model required quarterly participation with the *BridgeUp Impact Network*, comprised of all partner organizations. Working with the University of Houston's All Kids Alliance, the Impact Network convened the group to discuss challenges and successes to better align and amplify the work by the individual organizations. Together with these thought partners, the Impact Network served as a shared learning community, with instruction and information about how best to achieve continuous quality improvement and address sustainability and scalability challenges.

The BridgeUp leadership team maintained regular, continuous communication and hosted events, including the quarterly Impact Network gatherings, before, during, and after COVID-19. The remote events lacked the networking capability but served as a place for partners to share with colleagues the many challenges and opportunities experienced throughout the pandemic.

Relationships improved among teachers, administrators, and behavioral health providers due to regular partnership meetings. At Galveston ISD, the district program leaders, counselors, and behavioral health partners met on a monthly basis. They worked together to develop a referral system for students who needed behavioral health supports and services. The result was much stronger relationships between the schools and the providers.

During Phase II, partners were required to meet regularly and review Logic Model and Rapid Cycle Improvement data. This worked especially well because they could do midcourse corrections and adjust aspects of the BridgeUp implementation before the end of the semester. Because of these data meetings, they were able to make decisions about improvements to the programs. For example, a nonprofit working with one of the lowest ranked high schools in the region created a software data system to track student attendance, behavior, and coursework. Each school team met weekly to review the data. Students with poor attendance, frequent behavioral referrals, and/or failing grades were flagged. The team was able to determine what support and programming the student needed and tracked them on a weekly basis.

8.3 Examples of Challenges in Operations

Over the 7-year period of the BridgeUp project, there were several social, political, and natural disaster events that occurred externally to the functioning of the BridgeUp Center. The original gift to Menninger from the David and Helen Gurley Brown Trust/Helen Gurley Brown Foundation was irrevocable and nontransferrable. In our experience, this was an important lesson in funding, since unexpected changes in leadership can happen. When leadership changes, if there are not legal protections, there can be threats to the viability of the project.

Public health is always political, but more so during national crises, such as national weather disasters or pandemics, or when new, significant health or education legislation is passed. During BridgeUp's 7-year history, five serious events affected the implementation of the model.

1. The first challenge emerged soon after the final touches were completed on the BridgeUp model research and design. The BridgeUp leadership team members were connected to a large mental health school-based network. Immediately before the model and the RFP were disseminated to groups such as this one, there was an opportunity to speak with a Texas Education Agency board member about the model. The board member's response was that any hint of social and emotional learning (SEL) programming in schools would never happen in Texas public schools. In contrast, several states, including Illinois and California, were intentionally including SEL in the school day for kids from pre-K through 12th grade. Opponents believed that mental health, including emotional and social development, was something that should not be taught in schools and instead

belonged in the home or religious settings. This conversation may have restricted the model design, except for what happened a few weeks later on the national level.

2. The second development was a positive one for the BridgeUp launch. The rollout for the RFP process was scheduled for February 2016. The timeline was set before the uncanny timing of the *No Child Left Behind* (NCLB, 2001) act being replaced with *Every Student Succeeds Act* (ESSA) (U.S. Department of Education 2015). ESSA opened the door in public schools to include noncognitive instruction, as well as the traditional focus on cognitive teaching. Even though the Act was not officially implemented until 2017, SEL conversations began to emerge in Texas.
3. The third significant factor occurred with the beginning of the second academic year in August 2017, when Hurricane Harvey dumped over 50″ of rainwater on 10,000 square miles of Southeast Texas and Louisiana, exceeding the previous 1899 record by 62% (The Texas Standard, 2021). The hurricane caused trauma for students and school staff that were both directly and indirectly affected. Partners requested additional support, especially for behavioral and mental health services. Fortunately, BridgeUp had funding in reserve to cover these costs. Thousands of families were displaced, and much to the dismay of the BridgeUp partners, many schools delayed the opening of the fall semester. BridgeUp was committed to continuous quality improvement and encouraged both open dialog and midcourse corrections as needed. Examples of how some of these challenges were met in various ways, including, for example, surveys, were sent to the partners to assess their challenges with program implementation after the hurricane. As a result, programming and scheduling aspects were modified as needed.
4. Some of the BridgeUp schools had extensive damage from the floods. This disaster coincided with new research identifying increased prevalence of adolescent mental health disorders. Hurricane Harvey pales in concern, however, to the COVID-19 pandemic, which in no uncertain terms created a paradigm shift in the public's understanding of public health. In response to COVID-19, the BridgeUp leadership team convened remotely and engaged in scenario planning, with a public health focus (see, e.g., Neiner et al., 2004). These planning sessions were made easier due to the completion of a BridgeUp 3-year strategic planning document. In a short period of time, there were multiple scenarios outlined, all with the same goal: Keep the BridgeUp model active *remotely* in the schools during the 2020 spring school semester. One of the concrete recommendations included the reallocation of funding to help schools and families with technology needs.
5. The fifth primary challenge to the implementation began during the last academic year for the BridgeUp project, at the end of 2021. Anxious, depressed, stressed, and suicidal young people were caught up in a system of compassion-fatigued teachers, administrators, and mental health providers. The constant communication during the pandemic helped to inform the BridgeUp leadership that another reallocation of funding needed to expand mental health services for the adults working with the students.

8.4 Implementation Funding

As mentioned in a previous case study chapter, the BridgeUp Center, the development of the BridgeUp model, and the school-based programs were funded with a generous gift to The Menninger Clinic from the David and Helen Gurley Brown Trust, now the Helen Gurley Brown Foundation (HGB) in New York. The Menninger Clinic, located in Houston, Texas, is a nationally ranked leader in psychiatry.

Funding for all 7 years included most of the salary supports for BridgeUp and partnership leaders, grants, model design, development, training and testing, and mental health services. During Phase I, as the projects ramped up, funding covered training, technology, and evaluation. In Phase II, funding included professional development, innovation, remote technology for schools, and additional discretionary funding related to hardships such as Hurricane Harvey and COVID-19. Funding for the 7-year project was specifically designated to improve the mental health of vulnerable adolescents in the greater Houston area. The funding was invested in the community, schools, and nonprofits in order to design, develop, implement, and test the BridgeUp model, which serves as the demonstration project for the APMH model. Planning for interruptions such as natural disasters should be a part of the annual funding budget. The BridgeUp model was tested in a variety of schools and school districts, ranging from a total of 800 students in the smallest school to 50,000 students in the largest independent school district. Approximately 80% of the students were disadvantaged, and many of the schools were located in low-resourced schools and/or urban areas. The total number of students served over the 6-year period was 63,325, resulting in a total cost per student at $117.62 or $19.60 per student per year.

BridgeUp at Menninger postponed the FY2021 RFP process due to the uncertainty around school closings and quarantine extensions. Instead, in June 2020, we offered current, eligible grantees the opportunity to apply for Bridge funding for the 2020 fall semester. Given the stress and anxiety from COVID-19 and the growing racial and political unrest, trauma-informed practices were a priority for the next semester. BridgeUp identified a few great resources for schools, and Menninger clinicians continued to offer online workshops on topics such as trauma, anxiety, and suicide prevention.

8.4.1 Matching Grants for Magic Grant Recipients

Additionally, in Phase II, BridgeUp leadership partnered with Rice University's Center for Philanthropy and Nonprofit Leadership to work with each of the partners to build capacity in how best to achieve sustainability of the BridgeUp project in the schools. Significant matching funding was obtained from Texas philanthropic organizations. Two long-term grantees were selected to receive funding of $800,000 each, over a period of 5 years, from the Hogg Foundation for Mental Health. The purpose of the grants was to conduct community needs assessments and implement community-based mental health services. Additionally, a BridgeUp school district received $7,500,000 from a local foundation to implement the BridgeUp model in every school in the district. Their grants, totaling $9,100,000, build on BridgeUp partnerships and programs.

According to the Substance Abuse and Mental Health Services Administration (SAMHSA), in 2019, mental health spending accounted for only about 5.5% of overall national health spending. The World Economic Forum reported in 2021 that global funding for mental health is around 2%, with only 0.5% of philanthropic giving (World Economic Forum, 2021).

In October, 2023, Mindful Philanthropy issued a Call to Action for Philanthropy in the USA to increase private investment to $35 billion annually to address mental health, addiction, and well-being (Mindful Philanthropy, 2023). In a companion piece, this group published a road map for strategic investment (Mindful Philanthropy, n.d.). This report identifies five priority areas for collective philanthropic investment, and one of the areas includes "youth and their support systems," with intention to expand school-based support.

Menninger changed their charity care and community benefit allocation in 2018 so that eligible adolescents who needed significant mental health supports could be referred for care. Of the 110 students referred, 36 received lifesaving care. The costs were incurred partially through pre-allocated BridgeUp funding. Those families who qualified for financial assistance were eligible to receive treatment at no cost.

8.5 Examples of Challenges in Operations: COVID-19

As mentioned above, there were numerous challenges with the implementaion, especially during Phase I, yet clearly the effect of COVID-19 was the most significant challenge. As soon as the pandemic was declared on March 11, 2020, BridgeUp acted quickly on one of seven scenarios, which included increased engagement and support with nonprofit and school partners. Acting early, the grantees were able to shift the BridgeUp model implementation to virtual delivery, resulting in continuous service throughout the remainder of the school semester.

BridgeUp maintained constant communication and responded to grantees' needs accordingly. This enhanced communication with the many partners continued throughout the end of the pandemic. In the 2020 spring semester, BridgeUp surveyed partner schools about the impact of COVID-19. For children living in poverty or low-income communities, COVID-19 had devastating effects (Harman, n.d.). Top needs for students and their families were basic ones such as food and rent, technology for remote school, and mental health and emotional needs. BridgeUp responded with a portion of grant funds to be redirected for basic needs or technology. One school district delivered groceries and toiletries to families that were struggling to meet basic needs. They helped 39 students in BridgeUp schools, reaching a total 180 household members. Another partner surveyed students about their feelings throughout the COVID-19 spring of 2020 quarantine. Students reported high rates of stress, loneliness, anxiety, and also hope and gratefulness. Box 8.4 reflects a few student quotes (BridgeUp 2016–2022 Unpublished reports).

Box 8.4: Student Reflections During COVID-19 Quarantine (verbatim)

- "what has made me feel lonely is that I dont really have anyone to talk to as much as i do at school."
- "I feel very stressed and anxious because I feel like I cant do nothing all I do is be in my room 24/7."
- "What has made me feel this positive feelings is being able to live this hard moments with the people i love (but i do miss my friends A LOT)."

These periodic surveys from BridgeUp helped to inform the project directors about how best to redirect SEL content and the MTSS protocol.

8.6 Conclusions

This overview of the lessons learned from the demonstration project included learnings from what worked well and what needed improvement. Considerations of these examples speak to the development, implementation, growth and sustainability of successful mult-sector projects. All aspects require an ongoing cycle of analysis, reflection and adjustment. Building on success and learning from miscalculations is necessary and critical. Integrating the SEL programming with MTSS school-wide proved to be challenging, especially in the larger middle and high schools during Phase I of the BridgeUp implementation. In addition, there were varying levels of successful collaboration among partners. One of the challenges with the CI framework was the difficulty moving operations from silos to multisector partnerships that required joint decision-making. However, programs that were funded for multiple years and with strong leadership thrived.

During Phase II, the operations and programming worked seamlessly until COVID-19. However, most of the partners had 3–4 years of experience working with the BridgeUp model, and the shift to remote schooling worked well operationally. The challenges changed from operational issues to the mental health of students, teachers, administrators, and families.

After interviewing the three school districts 2 years after the BridgeUp project ended, their district-wide scalability and sustainability is the best measure of success for the model and brings confidence to the aspirational adolescent public mental health model that is proposed in this volume.

Competing Interests

1. The BridgeUp at Menninger study was generously funded by the David and Helen Gurley Brown Trust, BridgeUp: Mental Health at The Menninger Clinic.
2. Patricia Gail Bray *has received consultant fees from* The Menninger Clinic, located in Houston, Texas.

References

AAP (American Academy of Pediatrics). (2021). *Declaration of a national emergency in child and adolescent mental health*. Retrieved January 25, 2023, from https://www.aap.org/en/advocacy/child-and-adolescent-healthy-mental-development/aap-aacap-cha-declaration-of-a-national-emergency-in-child-and-adolescent-mental-health/

BridgeUp at Menninger. (2016–2022). Unpublished evaluations reports.

CASEL. (2019). *Connecting schoolwide SEL with other school-based frameworks*. Retrieved May 16, 2024, from https://schoolguide.casel.org/uploads/2019/01/SEL_MTSS-and-PBIS.pdf

Durlak, J. A., Domitrovich, C. E., Weissberg, R. P., & Gullotta, T. P. (2015). *Handbook of social and emotional learning: Research and practice*. https://ci.nii.ac.jp/ncid/BB19322885

Harman, L. (n.d.). *Coronavirus is a devastating blow to children in poverty*. Save the Children on behalf of the Global Coalition to End Child Poverty. Retrieved May 19, from https://www.savethechildren.org/us/charity-stories/effects-coronavirus-on-children-poverty

Institute of Medicine. (1994). In P. J. Mrazek & R. J. Haggerty (Eds.), *Reducing risks for mental disorder: Frontiers for preventive intervention research*. National Academy of Sciences.

Kania, J., & Kramer, M. (2011, Winter). Collective impact. *Stanford Social Innovation Review*. https://ssir.org/articles/entry/collective_impact

Kessler, R. C., Berglund, P. A., Demler, O. V., Jin, R., Merikangas, K. R., & Walters, E. E. (2005). Lifetime prevalence and age-of-onset distributions of DSM-IV disorders in the National Comorbidity Survey Replication. *Archives of General Psychiatry, 62*(6), 593. https://doi.org/10.1001/archpsyc.62.6.593

Lee, H. (1960). *To kill a Mockingbird*. J.B Lippincott & Co.

McGill, E., Er, V., Penney, T., et al. (2021). Evaluation of public health interventions from a complex systems perspective: A research methods review. *Social Science & Medicine, 272*. https://doi.org/10.1016/j.socscimed.2021.113697

Mindful Philanthropy. (2023). *Mental health at the center: A call to action for philanthropy*. Retrieved May 2, 2024, from https://www.mindfulphilanthropy.org/atthecenter

Mindful Philanthropy. (n.d.). *Mental health at the center: A roadmap for strategic investment*. Retrieved May 2, 2024, from https://virtuous-email.s3.amazonaws.com/Email/org_1872/Roadmap%20to%20Strategic%20Investment%20-%20Final.pdf

Neiner, J. A., Howze, E. H., & Greaney, M. L. (2004). Using scenario planning in public health: Anticipating alternative futures. *Health Promotion Practice*, 5(1), 69–79. Retrieved May 2, 2024, from https://doi.org/10.1177/1524839903257692.

No Child Left Behind Act (NCLB) of 2001. (2001). 20 U.S.C. § 6301 *et.seq.* https://www.congress.gov/bill/107th-congress/house-bill/1/text

O'Connell, M. E., Boat, T., & Warner, K. E., (Eds.). (2009). Preventing mental, emotional, and behavioral disorders among young people: Progress and possibilities. National Research Council (US) and Institute of Medicine (US) Committee on the prevention of mental disorders and substance abuse among children, youth, and young adults: Research advances and promising interventions, Washington, DC: National Academies Press (US). Retrieved January 12, 2023, from https://www.ncbi.nlm.nih.gov/books/NBK32775/pdf/Bookshelf_NBK32775.pdf

Simonsen, B., Robbie, K., Meyer, K., Freeman, J., Everett, S., & Feinberg A. (2021, November). Multi-tiered system of supports (MTSS) in the classroom. Center on PBIS, University of Oregon. Retrieved May 8, 2024, from www.pbis.org

The Texas Standard. (2021, February 10). Retrieved January 12, 2023. *Fact check: Did more water fall during Hurricane Harvey than during a year at Niagara Falls?* Retrieved January 12, 2023, from https://www.texasstandard.org/stories/fact-check-did-more-water-fall-during-hurricane-harvey-than-during-a-year-at-niagara-falls/

U.S. Department of Education. Every Student Succeeds Act. (2015). Retrieved January 12, 2023, from https://www.ed.gov/essa?src%3Drn

World Economic Forum. (2021). *How philanthropy could help provide better mental health care*. Retrieved April 6, 2024, from https://www.weforum.org/agenda/2021/07/how-philanthropy-could-help-provide-better-mental-health-care/

Chapter 9
Lessons, Part II: Barriers to Care

Oana Smaranda Pop

9.1 Introduction

BridgeUp at Menninger enabled students at affiliated schools to be referred to the Menninger Clinic for treatment. However, only a small fraction of referred students followed through with scheduling and attending their appointments. Though all individuals face barriers to accessing healthcare, the young people served by BridgeUp appeared to face more barriers than the average individual, preventing them from ultimately receiving the care they needed. The purpose of this literature review is to provide a better understanding of adolescents' barriers to accessing and obtaining mental and behavioral healthcare, specifically for those located in urban environments.

BridgeUp's mission was critical in ameliorating the health and wellness of local adolescents. Since the 1940s, the constitution of the World Health Organization has included fostering mental health as a key function of the organization (Constitution of the World Health Organization, 1946). There are complicated comorbidities between mental health conditions and communicable/noncommunicable diseases, and mental health has been found to impact disease prognosis as well (Prince et al., 2007). Improving mental health is, consequently, a requirement in improving overall health and wellness; the WHO has even stated "there can be no health without mental health" (WHO, 2005).

Mental health is crucial in the development of youth into their adulthood. Mental well-being involves a "positive sense of identity, the ability to manage thoughts, emotions, as well as to build relationships… enabling their full active participation in society" (WHO, 2013). Therefore, in order to ensure successful delivery of

O. S. Pop (✉)
Brown Fellow, BridgeUp at Menninger (formerly affiliated), The Menninger Clinic, Houston, TX, USA
e-mail: opop@berkeley.edu

P. G. Bray, A. Maerlender (eds.), *Adolescent Public Mental Health*,
https://doi.org/10.1007/978-3-031-68294-0_9

services to this population, BridgeUp needed to identify and overcome barriers specific to diverse adolescents in Greater Houston, and future projects must identify barriers within their own environments as well. This review sought to begin the former: identification of barriers for urban adolescents.

9.2 Definitions

9.2.1 *Mental Health*

According to the World Health Organization, mental health is "a state of well-being in which the individual realizes his or her own abilities, can cope with the normal stresses of life, can work productively and fruitfully, and is able to make a contribution to his or her community" (WHO, 2004). The National Institute of Mental Health (NIMH) broadly defines mental illness as a mental, behavioral, or emotional disorder—this includes conditions that cause symptoms and impairments ranging from mild to severe (2023).

Generally, the term "mental health" acts as an inclusive term for an individual's psychological and behavioral health. The semantics of defining mental health can be tenuous. Mental health can be fluid and dependent on individual context and culture, as described by Galderisi et al. (2015) and Galderisi (2024). This definition recognizes that emotions such as anger, sadness, and fear are a normal part of life, but a healthy individual can adapt to these fluctuations and maintain their internal equilibrium (Galderisi, 2024).

9.2.2 *Behavioral Health*

The Substance Abuse and Mental Health Services Administration, or SAMHSA, defines behavioral health as an intersection of mental health and resilience with the treatment of mental and substance use disorders, along with support from family and community (SAMHSA, n.d.). The consideration of substance use is critical in treating the whole individual's body and mind. A broad definition of behavioral healthcare is the "prevention, diagnosis, and treatment of [mental health and substance use disorders, life stressors and crises, and stress-related physical symptoms]" (American Medical Association, 2022).

9.2.3 *Conduct Disorder*

Conduct disorders are a contentious issue, with medical experts disagreeing on their underlying causes and classification. Conduct disorders are characterized as psychiatric conditions in which an afflicted individual repeatedly behaves in a manner that is not appropriate or respectful of other individuals' basic rights and/or behaviors that are not appropriate for one's age or social environment (Pisano et al., 2017). Behavior or conduct problems are multifaceted and complex, but early treatment can be effective (CDC, 2023).

9.2.4 Healthcare Access

Healthcare access is the timely entry and use of services to achieve optimal health outcomes for an individual, group of individuals, or community (Millman, 1993). Adequate access involves coverage of care, services provided, timeliness of care, and the healthcare workforce (Chartbook on Access to Health Care, n.d.).

9.2.5 Barriers to Accessing Care

Barriers prevent individuals or groups from adequately accessing and utilizing services. These can generally be categorized into supply-side and demand-side barriers.

Supply-side barriers prevent access due to factors innate to the healthcare system, which impede an individual or community from using a service (Jacobs et al., 2011). An example of a supply-side barrier is a lack of accessible clinics in rural regions compared to urban locations (AHRQ, 2023).

Demand-side barriers directly inhibit an individual's or community's ability to access and use a service (Jacobs et al., 2011). An example of a demand-side barrier is lack of insurance coverage, which is higher for some populations compared to others (AHRQ, 2023).

Besides supply and demand categorization, other barrier classifications exist. In a 2002 study, parents classified barriers into three major categories (Owens et al., 2002):

- Structural barrier, e.g., distance from service provider
- Perceptions about mental health problems, e.g., parental perception that problems should be handled at home
- Perceptions about mental health services, e.g., parental perception that previous experience with professionals was negative

In a different study focusing on individuals suffering from mental health conditions comorbid with substance use disorders, barriers were classified into two categories: personal characteristics barriers and structural barriers (Priester et al., 2016). Personal characteristics barriers were related to the patient's own vulnerabilities in treatment, and structural barriers were related to service provision, such as availability, location, and financial factors (Priester et al., 2016).

These differing classification methods demonstrate the complexity of targeting a specific barrier or class of barriers for intervention—"barriers" themselves are highly reliant on a provider's or public health professional's interpretation of barriers, the population of interest, and the context of an intervention.

9.2.6 Service Utilization

According to Andersen's behavioral model, service utilization is the *actual* usage of a service by an individual, family, household, or community (Andersen, 1995). The behavioral model frames service utilization as being modulated by predisposing, enabling, and needs factors. Predisposing factors increase an individual's or group's innate likelihood of utilizing services, and enabling factors make service access and utilization possible to achieve by the user (Andersen & Newman, 2005). Need is relative to the user's condition's severity—in order to seek services, there must be a perception that an illness or condition requires intervention and usually a professional's clinical decision that a service is indicated (Andersen & Newman, 2005).

9.2.7 Telemedicine

Telemedicine, broadly, is the use of technology or telecommunication to provide services remotely (Flodgren et al., 2015).

9.3 Epidemiology of Adolescent Mental Health

Studies show that there is a relatively high prevalence of mental illness among American adolescents; the 2001–2004 National Comorbidity Survey Adolescent Supplement estimated that 49.5% of adolescents had any mental disorder over their lifetime, while about 22% had a mental illness that caused severe impairment (NIMH, 2023). One CDC source estimated that as many as 20% of the children living in the USA experience mental health conditions in a year—a rate that is still increasing (Perou et al., 2013). However, since mental health is so broadly defined, it is necessary to delve into its components to truly understand how mental health impacts the younger population.

According to a 2019 study examining the prevalence of mental health, behavioral, and conduct problems among children ages 3–17, 6.1% of adolescents (ages 12–17) had a current diagnosis of depression, 10.5% had anxiety, and 7.5% had behavior/conduct problems (Ghandour et al., 2019). In metropolitan statistical areas and metropolitan principal cities, respectively, 2.8% and 3.6% had depression; 7.2% and 6.8% had anxiety; and 6.9% and 7.6% had behavior/conduct problems (Ghandour et al., 2019). The prevalence of these conditions is important for selecting priority populations and optimal interventions.

Physical conditions are often comorbid with psychological problems and vice versa. For example, people with mental health disorders suffer more from physical illness-related mortality than those without mental health disorders (WHO, 2013). In high income countries, at least 35% and up to 50% of people with severe mental health disorders do not receive treatment (WHO, 2013). Globally, mental, neurological, and substance use disorders compose 13% of the burden of disease, which is a considerable fraction.

Adolescents particularly have a high need for resources for mental and behavioral health—puberty and early adulthood are a life phase during which symptoms of psychiatric conditions tend to emerge, likely due to a combination of normal brain maturation with psychosocial and biological modulating factors (Paus et al., 2008). Between early adolescents (aged 11–12) and middle adolescents (13–14), research has found a marked increase in mental and behavioral health difficulties (Yoon et al., 2022). According to the WHO, "suicide is the second most common cause of death among young people worldwide" (2013). Texas—BridgeUp and Menninger's home state—ranks 35th in the USA for youth measures of mental health, indicating an elevated prevalence of health problems and low access to resources (Nguyen & Davis, 2017). 67.3% of youth in Texas who had experienced a major depressive episode had an unmet need for care, while 11.4% of youth did not have insurance that covered mental healthcare (Nguyen & Davis, 2017). This data illustrates the high need for programs such as BridgeUp, as well as organizations like Menninger, subsidizing care for those from low-income backgrounds.

9.4 Methods

A literature search was conducted using the keywords "barriers," "service utilization," "urban," "adolescent," and "health disparities," among others. Based on the results of searching in a variety of databases, it became clear that there was not a defined set of barriers to care that the urban adolescents face. Rather, barriers are very specific to the individual. An individual's race, ethnicity, gender, socioeconomic status, and current and past health problems modulate the individual's desire and ability to access care. Furthermore, for adolescents, parents or guardians face barriers of their own, which can subsequently impact the adolescent's access to care, regardless of their own attitudes. Findings from the literature are tabulated in Appendix A (Table 9.1) and categorized and described in the next sections.

9.5 Barriers

9.5.1 Race and Ethnicity

Race is a well-known social determinant of health and appears to permeate mental health service access and provision as well. A 2001 report by the surgeon general found that racial and ethnic minorities utilize mental health services at a significantly lower rate than their white counterparts and disproportionately less in relation to the prevalence of mental health conditions (HHS, 2001). According to this report, the "organization and financing of services" have created barriers for these communities, as well as stigma, discrimination, and mistrust of providers and services. Published research supports these conclusions.

In a 2008 study, black, Native American, and Hispanic children in urban areas reported higher rates of mental health problems compared to white children (Howell & McFeeters, 2008). However, Native American children had mental health visits at a statistically significantly higher rate than white children, and Hispanic children had a much lower rate than white children (Howell & McFeeters, 2008). Interestingly, Native American youths in Oregon were found to utilize mental health services less frequently than white youths, regardless of Medicaid status, indicating a racial disparity among this population (Deck & Vander Ley, 2006). Urban-located black children had fewer mental health visits than their white counterparts, although this was not statistically significant (Howell & McFeeters, 2008). Families of children belonging to minority racial groups tend to prefer informal sources of help as opposed to professional medical intervention (McKay et al., 1996). This may be a cultural preference or could reflect discrimination in healthcare, discouraging these groups to pursue certain services.

Finally, Hispanic children have a higher unmet need than white children due to racial disparities in accessing and receiving mental healthcare (Kataoka et al., 2002). A scarcity of bilingual mental health providers may contribute to this disparity and drive Hispanic families away from mental health services.

9.5.2 Gender

One study found that over the course of adolescence, females' mental health markedly deteriorated while males' stayed the same (Yoon et al., 2022). Female children were more likely than male children to attend at least one mental healthcare appointment, though adult women reportedly preferred certain treatment characteristics, such as empathetic, warm staff; client-directed goals; and female-only group therapy (McKay et al., 1996; Priester et al., 2016). Lacking these factors and options may deter adolescent girls from attending their appointments (Priester et al., 2016). Adolescent females were found to exhibit more help-seeking behaviors, although both females and males held similar attitudes toward help-seeking (De Luca et al., 2019). Females also seemed to have more trust in older individuals to provide help (De Luca et al., 2019), suggesting adolescent males might feel more helpless. In research with male-only study populations, help-seeking behaviors were perceived as a sign of weakness (Radez et al., 2021). Other studies found that men have lower utilization, possibly associated with gender roles and traditional views of masculinity (Chandra & Minkovitz, 2006). Thus, adolescent males seem to face more demand-side barriers, while females may face barriers on both supply and demand sides.

9.5.3 Socioeconomic Status

Barriers related to socioeconomic status (SES) were attributed to lack of insurance and inability to pay. These were found to potentially lead to higher incidence of co-occurring disorders for adolescents with low SES (Priester et al., 2016). Patients with low income were more likely to use emergency services or inpatient care for mental health treatment as opposed to outpatient mental healthcare (Zahner et al., 1992, qtd. in McKay et al., 1996). Barriers related to SES also included inconvenient clinic hours, long wait times for appointments, a requirement of multiple intake appointments before treatment, inability to maintain standing weekly appointments, stigma of mental health and poverty, mistrust and negative experiences with mental health providers, and parental apprehension of being separated from their children (Hodgkinson et al., 2017; Ofonedu et al., 2017). Families of children with low socioeconomic status may then rely on their own coping skills and informal supports, instead of professional mental healthcare.

For children with low socioeconomic status, one viable option is to receive services from school-based providers, if they are available. However, this comes with its own barriers—a 2013 study found that when mental health and academics were intertwined, teacher perceptions became a potential barrier, because they perceived mental healthcare as inessential to a student's academic success and well-being, albeit desirable (Schwean & Rodger, 2013). Teacher perceptions could create unintended barriers for adolescents to receive school-based care.

9.5.4 Current Illness, Disorder, or Health Condition

There is evidence that an adolescent's actual mental health or behavioral health condition can impact the barriers they experience in accessing or utilizing services. Children with illnesses scoring more severely on the Child Behavior Checklist[1] (Achenbach, n.d.) were more likely to receive treatment than their counterparts with less clinical need (Garland et al., 1996, qtd. in Burns et al., 2004). There may be an unmet need among children with low scores on the Child Behavior Checklist, if their providers deprioritize their care by using this particular metric.

Conversely, Priester et al. (2016) found that individuals with co-occurring disorders had lower usage of services than individuals not suffering from comorbid disorders—the authors suggested that there was a lack of specialized services catering to those with comorbid mental health and substance use disorders. There are also barriers specific to adolescents with co-occurring mental health conditions and substance use, such as disjointed care systems and fear of substance use being disclosed

[1]The Child Behavioral Checklist is a tool completed by caregivers and used by providers to help diagnose mental health and behavioral problems in children and adolescents (Achenbach, n.d.).

to parents (Sterling et al., 2010). It is possible that adolescents with these conditions are less likely to access and use services due to barriers on both the supply and demand side.

9.5.5 Psychiatric and Medical History

There is also evidence that an adolescent's history of psychiatric and mental healthcare can impact their access and use of services. It is important to distinguish that these barriers arise from an individual's *past* diagnoses, and not the condition for which they currently seek care.

Children who had received mental health services in sixth grade had lower odds of reporting barriers than their counterparts who had not received treatment (Owens et al., 2002). Similarly, children involved with the criminal justice system were more likely to attend intake appointments than those without a history of incarceration (McKay et al., 1996). In research where the study population comprised adolescents with a history of mental health issues, there was a preference for "rely[ing] on themselves" as opposed to professional help (Radez et al., 2021). Their past experiences with mental healthcare and institutions in the past may have differentially impacted their current abilities to access and receive care. This was also evident for children in the foster care system (see Sects. 9.5.6 "Influence of Parents" and 9.5.7 "Special Populations"). For families of children who had received care in the past, perceived barriers were related to their fear of being labeled or "medicalization" by teachers if the school had become involved in the child's healthcare (Fazel et al., 2014).

Children with histories of severe abuse and trauma were found to be more likely to attend intake appointments than children with aggressive or ADHD-related behaviors (McKay et al., 1996). Nevertheless, for survivors of trauma, barriers included hesitance to revisit traumatic memories, self-doubt, and not believing in their own need for help (Truss et al., 2023). Adolescents with a history of trauma still face the same structural barriers to mental healthcare as those without trauma (Ellinghaus et al., 2020) but evidently need additional supports in accessing care.

9.5.6 Influence of Parents

One of the most powerful determinants of an adolescent's access to care is their family—parents play a major role in their child's mental health and care history. Reardon et al. (2017) found four themes salient in British parents' perceived barriers and facilitators to care:

- Systemic/structural issues, e.g., costs of services (including travel and lost wages), systems difficult to navigate, long waiting times for appointments, inaccessible location.

- Attitudes toward providers and treatment, e.g., lack of trusting relationship with empathetic provider, language barrier, desire to solve problem informally.
- Knowledge and understanding of mental health and help-seeking, e.g., lack of parental recognition of severity of child's condition.
- Family circumstances, e.g., poor familial support system, unable to make time commitment for treatment.

These themes are reflected in findings from other studies as well. For example, Owens et al. (2002) found that parents who claimed that their additional responsibilities limited their time had five times the odds of reporting structural barriers than their counterparts—an example of a family circumstances barrier. Additionally, parents who reported many stressors in daily life had significantly increased odds of reporting structural and stigma-related barriers, and divorced parents reported more stigma-related barriers (Owens et al., 2002). Family circumstances also impacted children living with foster caregivers—they were much more likely to attend appointments than children with a single mother as their primary caretaker (McKay et al., 1996).

In another British study, Sayal et al. (2010) reported parental barriers directly aligning with Reardon's systemic/structural issues, attitudes, and knowledge themes:

- Systemic/structural: Appointments were too short to present or address problems; practitioner had poor attitude.
- Attitudes: Parents were embarrassed or scared of child receiving a diagnosis.
- Knowledge: Parents didn't think behavioral problem was a real health problem; parents believed child's diagnosis would lead to judgment of their parenting and ultimately separation from their child.

These barriers are exemplified in a 2023 study on caregivers of adolescents hospitalized for psychiatric illness. In addition to the sheer stress brought on by having a loved one hospitalized, caregivers reported challenges such as lack of financial resources, feelings of embarrassment and stigma, and lack of support (D'Angelo et al., 2023).

Since parents of children and young adolescents are usually responsible for their care and, by extension, their medical treatment, barriers for parents effectively act as barriers for their children. Targeting parents whose children have a history of mental healthcare may prove to be extremely useful in increasing access and usage.

9.5.7 Special Populations

There are a number of special populations that merit attention for their unique lived experiences and cultural histories. Barriers for youth in foster care, in contact with the criminal justice system, and refugees have been studied.

Adolescents in foster care with mental health needs are a special population that should not be treated as equivalent to the general population of young people. For youth in foster care, type of foster placement played a role in utilizing care (Burns et al., 2004). Maltreatment by neglect was related to low service utilization (Burns et al., 2004). Receipt of care or services was also positively correlated to older age, indicating that younger age may act as a determinant of low utilization.

Adolescents who have been in contact with the criminal justice system represent a population with different needs and require different approaches to care. According to a 2009 study, parents of these children did not perceive behavioral problems as connected to mental health conditions and ascribed behaviors to family-related problems and traumas (Watson et al., 2009). The same study found that these families may have had poor experiences with care in the past, further contributing to their neutral or even negative perceptions of mental health conditions and mental healthcare.

Adolescents with refugee or immigrant backgrounds may have vastly different needs compared to those who were born and raised in the USA. In a 2015 study, eight themes were found to encompass refugees' barriers to accessing mental healthcare, including the following (Colucci et al., 2015):

- Trust and distrust: negative lived experiences with authority figures.
- Cultural concepts: cultural disconnect between provider and client.
- Engaging family/community: poor provider understanding of dynamics.

Furthermore, immigrants (whether noncitizens or naturalized) were found to be less likely to take medications and access mental health resources than US citizens (Chen & Vargas-Bustamante, 2011). Noncitizens were much more likely to be uninsured and less likely to receive regular care (Chen & Vargas-Bustamante, 2011). Language barriers, lack of primary care, and perceptions were reasons for low usage, aligning with Colucci et al.'s (2015) themes.

9.5.8 Potential Solutions

Potential solutions include methods to reduce barriers as well as research on increasing access and service utilization specific to certain demographics.

For youth and families with little past experience with mental health resources, existing research indicated that high engagement with parents augmented youth attendance of intake and other appointments. An intensely engaging phone call preceding intake appointments increased attendance by over 25% (McKay et al., 1996). Logistical support for families navigating mental health for the first time was found to build trusting relationships between families/youth and staff/providers (Reardon et al., 2017). Engaging with the whole family and engaging with youth in their day-to-day context were found to better address the social determinants of mental health and therefore helped providers better care for patients; addressing parents stress demonstrably improved outcomes for children receiving care (Hodgkinson et al., 2017; Kazdin & Whitley, 2003). These studies demonstrate that high engagement and guidance of families and youth can augment their experiences with mental healthcare and consequently improve outcomes.

For refugees, Colucci et al. (2015) described barrier-specific solutions such as a provider understanding and respect toward the patient's culture, with the goal of building a trusting relationship with patients with different cultural backgrounds and a possible history of trauma. For other special populations like youth in contact with the criminal justice system, Burns et al. (2004) suggested more provider education and improving collaboration between institutions like the criminal justice system, welfare systems, and mental health providers.

The concept of continuity of care arose in numerous studies and provides a generalizable course of action for minimizing barriers, not only for special populations. School-based mental health services could improve continuity of care for those unable to afford treatment and could help overcome financial barriers (Schwean & Rodger, 2013). Educating families about trauma and improving continuity of care were also shown to improve access and usage (Sayal et al., 2010; Damian et al., 2018). Finally, for situations in which continuity of care is not achievable, solutions like telemedicine can come into play to best serve the community (Fazel et al., 2014).

In addition to directly targeting known barriers, continuing research on service access and utilization would provide valuable information on the behavioral and psychological foundations of mental health access. Existing research has shown that needs factors were significant predictors of service utilization (Fleury et al., 2014; Dey & Jorm, 2017). This research provides a foundation for future research on mental health service utilization of urban youth.

9.5.9 Synthesis in Context

Existing research provided a large quantity of information on the barriers to access that BridgeUp referral patients likely faced when seeking services at the Menninger Clinic. Notably, the adolescents whom BridgeUp served were fundamentally different from the population that Menninger had catered to in the past. BridgeUp referrals and their families may have had little to no mental health literacy. While usual Menninger patients would have sought out care specifically at this Clinic, BridgeUp adolescents had to be referred there, and in most cases the campus was far away from the students' local community. Additional resources and attention needed to be provided to ensure BridgeUp adolescents' entry and usage of the care—more engaging interactions were needed from staff and providers. Future programs and interventions must not generalize adolescents into the broader population of care-seeking individuals.

The volume of these findings did not completely elucidate the issue of barriers to care. While considerable research focuses on access to care by rural populations, there appears to be a paucity of scientific inquiry into adolescents located in urban settings, so additional questions arose during review of existing literature.

- When is parental involvement appropriate? Could parental involvement/participation be a barrier in certain situations?

- It might be in adolescents' best interests to receive care within their own community or with their existing primary care provider (Hodgkinson et al., 2017)—how do new programs and interventions navigate the responsibility to provide quality care best suited to populations of interest?
- If interventions are unable to completely resolve adolescents' barriers, who can? What are the next steps?

These questions provided an opportunity to reassess the role of programs like BridgeUp and institutions like Menninger within their communities' health. Telemedicine is one solution that can be harnessed to both overcome barriers and increase utilization.

9.6 Telemedicine

Using technology to provide mental healthcare can potentially resolve numerous barriers regardless of individual's demographics by overcoming some common barriers. Telemental health has been found to be as effective as in-person care, and it can also cater to specific populations and their unique barriers (Gloff et al., 2015). Telemedicine is worth exploring as an option for adolescents in urban settings.

9.6.1 Potential Benefits

Numerous studies have found that the use of technology in mental healthcare, or telemedicine/telemental healthcare, is popular among children and adolescents—they are comfortable with technology, it is generally an accessible tool, and they may find it fun and appealing (Boydell et al., 2010, 2014; Myers et al., 2010; Russo et al., 2017). Past studies found that teenagers were not only satisfied with technology but were also enthusiastic to use it for their mental healthcare (Grealish et al., 2005; Boydell et al., 2010). Among young adults, using technology promoted positive relationships with their providers (Boydell et al., 2014). Using technology decreased negative perceptions, stigma, and nervousness about attending appointments among youth, which were significant barriers to care (Boydell et al., 2010, 2014; Gloff et al., 2015). It also helped overcome language barriers by allowing patients to receive care in their native language without the need for an interpretation service (Di Carlo et al., 2021). Telemedicine may also be a critical tool in maintaining continuity of care for adolescents nearing adulthood as they age out of the school-based care safety net (Khetarpal et al., 2022).

Telemedicine also has numerous other measurable, barrier-reducing characteristics. Time-saving and cost-saving aspects may be attractive to parents of the individuals receiving care (Boydell et al., 2014; Russo et al., 2017). Studies found that although telemedicine has generally been implemented to increase access for rural communities, it is also useful for urban communities, since many of the same barriers are salient in both settings (Grubagh et al., 2008; Spaulding et al., 2011). Furthermore, during the COVID-19 pandemic, telemedicine was critical in maintaining continuity of care in the face of outbreak of a highly infectious disease (Di Carlo et al., 2021). The need for social distancing enabled telemedicine to demonstrate its practicality in situations where face-to-face care was not available or advisable (Whaibeh et al., 2020).

9.6.2 *Possible Problems*

Though telemedicine can reduce barriers, there are pitfalls. Technological difficulties arose as an issue in numerous studies, and this deficit was more pronounced for populations with low socioeconomic status (Boydell et al., 2014; Gloff et al., 2015). Another issue was the need for funds to be allocated toward the technology and therefore away from staffing, raising questions on the sustainability of this solution and responsibilities of the healthcare workforce (Grealish et al., 2005). Additionally, some states do not require insurance to cover all telemental health services—in 33 states, Medicaid solely covers audio-only telehealth for CHIP recipients (McBain et al., 2023).

Demand-side problems with telemedicine included parental lack of trust toward virtual care (Russo et al., 2017); a depersonalized patient experience; minimal trust established in the first appointment, which discouraged follow-up; and concerns about elopement, distraction, and privacy (Boydell et al., 2010; Di Carlo et al., 2021; Gloff et al., 2015; Inwards-Breland et al., 2024). Young patients seeking gender-affirming care also cited seeing themselves on camera as a disadvantage (Inwards-Breland et al., 2024). Clinicians were found to be more resistant to adopting telemedicine (Grealish et al., 2005; Di Carlo et al., 2021).

A final issue was that virtual treatment and diagnosis could be less accurate than in-person treatment, due to behavioral subtleties that may be lost in translation over virtual communication (Boydell et al., 2014; Di Carlo et al., 2021). Though high-bandwidth connections and quality cameras can remedy this gap (Gloff et al., 2015), the financial situation of the adolescent would determine whether these are accessible. These gaps must continue to be addressed in evidence-based, comparative research to determine the efficacy of telemedicine versus traditional face-to-face treatment.

9.7 Proposed Next Steps

Though the published research on barriers to care can be difficult to synthesize in the context of urban adolescents, there are actions that can reduce the barriers or at least make them easier to overcome. First, in general, there must be more research conducted specifically on minority populations located in urban areas. Additionally, qualitative research can glean useful information from key informants, including parents, school officials, and community healthcare providers. It is evident that numerous barriers can be overcome with the use of technology—it would be fruitful to consider implementing telemental health both in schools and by healthcare providers.

Much of the research evidence indicates that parental or guardian barriers play a major role in adolescents' own access to treatment. Since parents are generally financially responsible for their children's care, improving charity care access and outreach may reduce parental barriers and increase the access of adolescents to needed services.

Finally, it may be advisable to connect moderate-to-high-need adolescents with community providers who are more familiar with the adolescent's social context and who may be more accessible to children and parents. Bolstering community capabilities could provide a longer-term solution for connecting youth to consistent, accessible care.

9.8 Conclusion

It is apparent that adolescents in urban settings face numerous challenges in receiving mental or behavioral health treatment. Based on the actual experience of BridgeUp as well as published research, adolescents are at a disadvantage because their health problems are equally complex yet unlike those of adults. Youth from low-income or minority communities are doubly burdened by lack of outreach, poor institutional cultural awareness, and stigma. Also, large institutions with the most resources are disconnected from the surrounding community, despite a high level of need.

The Menninger Clinic is notable in that it provides treatment specific to adolescents. Numerous other institutions do not. Therefore, a major recommendation for urban service providers is to cater more specifically toward adolescents. This would not only allow for specialized treatment for adolescents but would increase the ability to engage their families in treatment and reduce caregiver-related barriers.

Institutions in large cities should conduct more in-depth needs assessments and community outreach to better understand the populations they serve. Cultural disconnect is a nuanced barrier when adolescents seek care; thus, improved cultural awareness among institutions and providers could combat it.

This literature review investigated broadly the barriers urban adolescents could face, but there is considerably more work to be done, ranging from within urban communities to the national policy landscape. While healthcare itself is considered a privilege by many, there must be increased efforts to ensure that adolescents receive equitable access to mental healthcare, regardless of their individual characteristics and life circumstances.

Competing Interests

1. *The BridgeUp at Menninger study was generously funded by the David and Helen Gurley Brown Trust, BridgeUp: Mental Health at The Menninger Clinic.*
2. *Oana Smaranda Pop has received consultant fees from The Menninger Clinic, located in Houston, Texas.*

Appendix A: Abstraction of Findings from Existing Research

Table 9.1 Barriers to care: abstraction of findings from existing research

Source	Population of interest	Barrier(s)	Supply/ demand side?
Burns et al. (2004)	Children with history of maltreatment	Low CBCL score Neglect (vs. sexual abuse) history African-American race Living at home	Supply
Chandra and Minkovitz (2006)	Eighth graders	Mental health knowledge Stigma Male gender (vs. female) Parental disapproval	Demand
Chen and Vargas-Bustamante (2011)	Patients with depression or anxiety disorders	Immigration status (vs. US-born)	Supply
Colucci et al. (2015)	Refugee youth	Lack of provider cultural humility Lack of provider understanding of illnesspoor accessibility Low provider trust Poor interpretation services Low family/community engagement Inappropriate provider style Lack of care continuity	Supply + demand
D'Angelo, Ofosu, and Preyde (2023)	Caregivers of youth hospitalized for psychiatric illness	Lack of financial resources Stigma Lack of support (social and institutional)	Supply + demand
Damian et al. (2018)	Youth with polytrauma or in contact with criminal justice system or welfare	Lack of care coordination Workforce shortage Socioeconomic constraints	Supply + demand
De Luca et al. (2019)	Central Texas adolescents	Male gender (vs. female)	Supply + demand
Deck and Vander Ley (2006)	Adolescents in Oregon	Medicaid eligibility Native American race Primary caretaker is parent (vs. foster)	Supply
Ellinghaus et al. (2020)	Trauma-exposed young people	Lack of trauma-informed care Cost Past negative experiences	Supply + demand
Fazel et al. (2014)	Children/adolescents in schools	Fear of "medicalization"	Demand
Garland et al. (1996)	Youth in foster care for ≤5 months	Neglect (vs. sexual/physical abuse) history Low clinical need History of passive (vs. active) maltreatment	Supply

(continued)

Table 9.1 (continued)

Source	Population of interest	Barrier(s)	Supply/ demand side?
HHS (2001)	Racial and ethnic minorities	Cost and lack of health insurance Fragmented services Culturally mediated stigma Mistrust of mental healthcare system Insensitivity of mental healthcare systems	Supply + demand
Hodgkinson et al. (2017)	Children and families living in poverty	African American or Hispanic (vs. white/non-Hispanic) Rural (vs. urban) location Distance from services Lack of insurance Lack of services provided under managed care plans Inconvenient/inflexible clinic hours Long wait times Multiple intake appointments required Stigma of mental healthcare Stigma of living in poverty Mistrust of mental healthcare system Provider bias against low-income families	Supply + demand
Howell and McFeeters (2008)	Children	Hispanic or black (vs. white/ non-Hispanic) Rural (vs. urban) location (Hispanic only)	Supply
Kataoka et al. (2002)	Children and adolescents	Hispanic (vs. non-Hispanic) Lack of insurance Younger age	Supply
McKay et al. (1996)	"Inner-city" youth	Male (vs. female) Primary caretaker is parent (vs. foster) More severe abuse/trauma Higher clinical need Older age	Supply + demand
Ofonedu et al. (2017)	Low-income racial/ethnic minority families	Living with 4+ people Parent suffering depression Delay between intake and treatment	Supply + demand
Owens et al. (2002)	Families of seventh graders in Baltimore, Maryland	Parenting difficulties Parental schedule constraints Parental stress Divorced parents Child's use of mental health services in the past Parent unemployment/disability	Demand

(continued)

Table 9.1 (continued)

Source	Population of interest	Barrier(s)	Supply/ demand side?
Priester et al. (2016)	Adults with co-occurring disorders (COD)	Lack of COD service availability Under identification of COD Lack of provider training on COD Insurance/financial barriers Non-white race	Supply + demand
Radez et al. (2021)	Children and adolescents	Limited mental health knowledge Perception of help-seeking Stigma Low trust Financial cost Logistical barriers	Supply + demand
Reardon et al. (2017)	Parents of children and adolescents with mental health need	Time limitations for family Poor family support system Bad past experiences with providers/treatment Low trust of mental health system Stigma Poor knowledge of process and problem Inefficient mental health system	Supply + demand
Sayal et al. (2010)	Parents of children with emotional or behavioral problems	Short appointment length Stigma Concerns about being labeled or diagnosed Fear of parent being judged and separated from child	Supply + demand
Schwean and Rodger (2013)	Canadian children and youth	Doubt that health services should be provided at school Perception of mental health as desirable but not essential Low community involvement Fragmented care Lack of regular services, follow-up, or communication	Supply
Sterling et al. (2010)	Adolescents with co-occurring disorders	Lack of integrated treatment options Lack of provider knowledge High cost of care Fear of substance use disclosure	Supply + demand
Truss et al. (2023)	Young people with trauma	Self-doubt, avoidance Fear and distrust of others	Demand
Watson et al. (2009)	Youth in criminal justice system with mental health needs	Stigma Lack of knowledge about mental health Low social support system	Supply + demand

References

Achenbach System of Empirically Based Assessment (ASEBA). (n.d.). *Child Behavior Checklist/6-18*. Retrieved from https://store.aseba.org/CHILD-BEHAVIOR-CHECKLIST_6-18/productinfo/201/. Accessed 10 Mar 2024.

Agency for Healthcare Research and Quality (AHRQ). (2023). *2023 National healthcare quality and disparities report*. Retrieved from https://www.ahrq.gov/research/findings/nhqrdr/nhqdr23/index.html. Accessed 10 Mar 2024.

American Medical Association. (2022). *What is behavioral health?* Retrieved from https://www.ama-assn.org/delivering-care/public-health/what-behavioral-health. Accessed 12 Mar 2024.

Andersen, R. M. (1995). Revisiting the behavioral model and access to medical care: Does it matter? *Journal of Health and Social Behavior, 36*, 1–10. https://doi.org/10.2307/2137284

Andersen, R. M., & Newman, J. F. (2005). Societal and individual determinants of medical care utilization in the United States. *Milbank Quarterly, 83*(4). https://doi.org/10.1111/2Fj.1468-0009.2005.00428.x

Boydell, K. M., Volpe, T., & Pignatiello, A. (2010). A qualitative study of young people's perspectives on receiving psychiatric services via televideo. *Journal of the Canadian Academy of Child and Adolescent Psychiatry, 19*(1), 5–11. https://www.ncbi.nlm.nih.gov/pmc/articles/PMC2809440/

Boydell, K. M., Hodgins, M., Pignatiello, A., Teshima, J., Edwards, H., & Willis, D. (2014). Using technology to deliver mental health services to children and youth: A scoping review. *Journal of the Canadian Academy of Child and Adolescent Psychiatry, 23*(2), 87–99. https://www.ncbi.nlm.nih.gov/pubmed/24872824

Burns, B. J., Phillips, S. D., Wagner, H. R., Barth, R. P., Kolko, D. J., Campbell, Y., & Landsverk, J. (2004). Mental health need and access to mental health services by youths involved with child welfare: A national survey. *Journal of the American Academy of Child and Adolescent Psychiatry, 43*(8), 960–970. https://doi.org/10.1097/01.chi.0000127590.95585.65

Centers for Disease Control and Prevention (CDC). (2023). *Behavior or conduct problems in children*. CDC: Children's Mental Health Disorders. Retrieved from https://www.cdc.gov/childrensmentalhealth/behavior.html. Accessed 10 Mar 2024

Chandra, A., & Minkovitz, C. S. (2006). Stigma starts early: Gender differences in teen willingness to use mental health services. *Journal of Adolescent Health, 38*(6), 754.e1. https://doi.org/10.1016/j.jadohealth.2005.08.011

Chartbook on Access to Health Care. (n.d.). *Agency for healthcare research and quality*. Retrieved from https://www.ahrq.gov/research/findings/nhqrdr/chartbooks/access/elements.html. Accessed 10 May 2024.

Chen, J., & Vargas-Bustamante, A. (2011). Estimating the effects of immigration status on mental health care utilizations in the United States. *Journal of Immigrant and Minority Health, 13*(4), 671–680. https://doi.org/10.1007/s10903-011-9445-x

Colucci, E., Minas, H., Szwarc, J., Guerra, C., & Paxton, G. (2015). In or out?: Barriers and facilitators to refugee-background young people accessing mental health services. *Transcultural Psychiatry, 52*(6), 766–790. https://doi.org/10.1177/1363461515571624

Constitution of the World Health Organization. (1946). *American Journal of Public Health, 36*(11), 1315–1323. https://doi.org/10.2105/AJPH.36.11.1315

D'Angelo, A., Ofosu, A., & Preyde, M. (2023). Adolescents hospitalized for psychiatric illness: Caregiver perspectives on challenges. *Adolescents, 3*(4), 651–666. https://doi.org/10.3390/adolescents3040046

Damian, A. K., Gallo, J. J., & Mendelson, T. (2018). Barriers and facilitators for access to mental health services by traumatized youth. *Children and Youth Services Review, 85*, 273–278. https://doi.org/10.1016/j.childyouth.2018.01.003

De Luca, S. M., Lim, J., & Yueqi, Y. (2019). Young adolescents' help seeking behaviors and attitudes: An examination of an underserved community. *Child and Adolescent Social Work Journal, 36*(6), 599–607. https://doi.org/10.1007/2Fs10560-019-00604-z

Deck, D., & Vander Ley, K. (2006). Medicaid eligibility and access to mental health services among adolescents in substance abuse treatment. *Psychiatric Services, 57*(2), 263–265. https://doi.org/10.1176/appi.ps.57.2.263

Dey, M., & Jorm, A. F. (2017). Social determinants of mental health service utilization in Switzerland. *International Journal of Public Health, 62*(1), 85–93. https://doi.org/10.1007/s00038-016-0898-5

Di Carlo, F., Sociali, A., Picutti, E., Pettorruso, M., Vellante, F., Verrastro, V., Martinotti, G., & di Giannantonio, M. (2021). Telepsychiatry and other cutting-edge technologies in COVID-19 pandemic: Bridging the distance in mental health assistance. *The International Journal of Clinical Practice, 75*(1), 10.1111.ijcp.13716.

Ellinghaus, C., Truss, K., Siling, J. L., Phillips, L., Eastwood, O., Medrano, C., & Bendall, S. (2020). "I'm tired of being pulled from pillar to post": A qualitative analysis of barriers to mental health care for trauma-exposed young people. *Early Intervention in Psychiatry, 15*(1), 113–122. https://doi.org/10.1111/eip.12919

Fazel, M., Hoagwood, K., Stephan, S., & Ford, T. (2014). Mental health interventions in schools in high-income countries. *The Lancet: Psychiatry, 1*(5), 377–387. https://doi.org/10.1016/S2215-0366(14)70312-8

Fleury, M. J., Ngui, A. N., Bamvita, J. M., Grenier, G., & Caron, J. (2014). Predictors of healthcare service utilization for mental health reasons. *International Journal of Environmental Research and Public Health, 11*(1), 10559–10586. https://doi.org/10.3390/ijerph111010559

Flodgren, G., Rachas, A., Farmer, A. J., Inzitari, M., & Shepperd, S. (2015). Interactive telemedicine: Effects on professional practice and health care outcomes. *Cochrane Database of Systematic Reviews, 9*, CD002098. https://doi.org/10.1002/14651858.CD002098.pub2

Galderisi, S. (2024). The need for a consensual definition of mental health. *World Psychiatry, 23*(1), 52–53. https://doi.org/10.1002/wps.21150

Galderisi, S., Heinz, A., Kastrup, M., Beezhold, J., & Sartorius, N. (2015). Toward a new definition of mental health. *World Psychiatry, 14*(2), 231–233. https://doi.org/10.1002/2Fwps.20231

Garland, A. F., Landsverk, J., Hough, R. L., & Ellis-Macleod, E. (1996). Type of maltreatment as a predictor of mental health service use for children in foster care. *Child Abuse and Neglect, 20*(8), 675–688. https://doi.org/10.1016/0145-2134(96)00056-7

Ghandour, R. M., Sherman, L. J., Vladutiu, C. J., Ali, M. M., Lynch, S. E., Bitsko, R. H., & Blumberg, S. J. (2019). Prevalence and treatment of depression, anxiety, and conduct problems in US children. *The Journal of Pediatrics, 206*, 256–267. https://doi.org/10.1016/j.jpeds.2018.09.021

Gloff, N. E., LeNoue, S. R., Novins, D. K., & Myers, K. (2015). Telemental health for children and adolescents. *International Review of Psychiatry, 27*(6), 513–524. https://doi.org/10.3109/09540261.2015.1086322

Grealish, A., Hunter, A., Glaze, R., & Potter, L. (2005). Telemedicine in a child and adolescent mental health service: Participants' acceptance and utilization. *Journal of Telemedicine and Telecare, 11*(Suppl. 1), 53–55. https://doi.org/10.1258/1357633054461921

Grubagh, A. L., Cain, G. D., Elhai, J. D., Patrick, S. L., & Frueh, B. C. (2008). Attitudes toward medical and mental health care delivered via telehealth applications among rural and urban primary care patients. *The Journal of Nervous and Mental Disease, 196*(2), 166–170. https://doi.org/10.1097/NMD.0b013e318162aa2d

Health and Human Services (HHS). (2001). *Mental health: Culture, race, and ethnicity—A supplement to mental health: A report of the surgeon general*. HHS, SAMHSA, Center for Mental Health Services. Retrieved from https://www.ncbi.nlm.nih.gov/books/NBK44243/. Accessed 10 May 2024

Hodgkinson, S., Godoy, L., Beers, L. S., & Lewin, A. (2017). Improving mental health access for low-income children and families in the primary care setting. *Pediatrics, 139*(1). https://doi.org/10.1542/peds.2015-1175

Howell, E., & McFeeters, J. (2008). Children's mental health care: Differences by race/ethnicity in urban/rural areas. *Journal of Health Care for the Poor and Underserved, 19*(1), 237–247. https://doi.org/10.1353/hpu.2008.0008

Inwards-Breland, D. J., Yeh, D., Marinkovic, M., Richardson, T. R., Marino-Kibbee, B., Bayley, A., & Rhee, K. E. (2024). Facilitators and barriers to using telemedicine for gender-affirming care in gender-diverse youth: A qualitative study. *Journal of Telemedicine and Telecare*. https://doi.org/10.1177/1357633X241231015

Jacobs, B., Ir, P., Bigdeli, M., Annear, P. L., & Van Damme, W. (2011). Addressing access barriers to health services: An analytical framework for selecting appropriate interventions in low-income Asian countries. *Health Policy and Planning, 27*(4), 288–300. https://doi.org/10.1093/heapol/czr038

Kataoka, S. H., Zhang, L., & Wells, K. B. (2002). Unmet need for mental health care among U.S. children: Variation by ethnicity and insurance status. *The American Journal of Psychiatry, 159*(9), 1548–1555. https://doi.org/10.1176/appi.ajp.159.9.1548

Kazdin, A. E., & Whitley, M. K. (2003). Treatment of parental stress to enhance therapeutic change among children referred for aggressive and antisocial behavior. *Journal of Consulting and Clinical Psychology, 71*(3), 504–515. https://doi.org/10.1037/0022-006x.71.3.504

Khetarpal, S. K., Auster, L. S., Miller, E., & Goldstein, T. R. (2022). Transition age youth mental health: Addressing the gap with telemedicine. *Child and Adolescent Psychiatry and Mental Health, 16*(1), 8. https://doi.org/10.1186/s13034-022-00444-3

McBain, R. K., Schuler, M. S., Qureshi, N., Matthews, S., Kofner, A., Breslau, J., & Cantor, J. H. (2023). Expansion of telehealth availability for mental health care after state-level policy changes from 2019 to 2022. *JAMA Network Open, 6*(6). https://doi.org/10.1001/2Fjamanetworkopen.2023.18045

McKay, M. M., McCadam, K., & Gonzales, J. J. (1996). Addressing the barriers to mental health services for inner city children and their caretakers. *Community Mental Health Journal, 32*(4), 353–361. https://doi.org/10.1007/BF02249453

Millman, M. (Ed.). (1993). *Access to health care in America*. National Academies Press.

Myers, K. M., Vander Stoep, A., McCarty, C. A., Klein, J. B., Palmer, N. B., Geyer, J. R., & Melzer, S. M. (2010). Child and adolescent telepsychiatry: Variations in utilization, referral patterns and practice trends. *Journal of Telemedicine and Telecare, 16*(3), 128–133. https://doi.org/10.1258/2Fjtt.2009.090712

National Institute of Mental Health (NIMH). (2023, March). *Mental illness*. . Retrieved from https://www.nimh.nih.gov/health/statistics/mental-illness.shtml. Accessed 10 Mar 2024.

Nguyen, T., & Davis, K. (2017). *The state of mental health in America 2017*. Mental Health America. Retrieved from http://www.mentalhealthamerica.net/sites/default/files/2017%20MH%20in%20America%20Full.pdf. Accessed 13 May 2019

Ofonedu, M. E., Belcher, H. M. E., Budhathoki, C., & Gross, D. A. (2017). Understanding barriers to initial treatment engagement among underserved families seeking mental health services. *Journal of Child and Family Studies, 26*(3), 863–876. https://doi.org/10.1007/2Fs10826-016-0603-6

Owens, P. L., Hoagwood, K., Horwitz, S. M., Leaf, P. J., Poduska, J. M., Kellam, S. G., & Ialongo, N. S. (2002). Barriers to children's mental health services. *Journal of the American Academy of Child and Adolescent Psychiatry, 41*(6), 731–738. https://doi.org/10.1097/00004583-200206000-00013

Paus, T., Keshavan, M., & Giedd, J. N. (2008). Why do many psychiatric disorders emerge during adolescence? *Nature Reviews: Neuroscience, 9*(12), 947–957. https://doi.org/10.1038/nrn2513

Perou, R., Bistko, R. H., Blumberg, S. J., Pastor, P., Ghandour, R. M., Gfroerer, J. C., Hedden, S. L., Crosby, A. E., et al. (2013). Mental health surveillance among children—United States, 2005–2011. *Morbidity and Mortality Weekly Report Supplements, 62*(02), 1–35. Retrieved from https://www.cdc.gov/mmwr/preview/mmwrhtml/su6202a1.htm. Accessed 10 Mar 2024

Pisano, S., Muratori, P., Gorga, C., Levantini, V., Iuliano, R., Catone, G., Coppola, G., Milone, A., & Masi, G. (2017). Conduct disorders and psychopathy in children and adolescents: Aetiology, clinical presentation and treatment strategies of callous-unemotional traits. *Italian Journal of Pediatrics, 43*(1), 84. https://doi.org/10.1186/s13052-017-0404-6

Priester, M. A., Browne, T., Iachini, A., Clone, S., DeHart, D., & Seay, K. D. (2016). Treatment access barriers and disparities among individuals with co-occurring mental health and substance use disorders: An integrative literature review. *Journal of Substance Abuse Treatment, 61*, 47–59. https://doi.org/10.1016/j.jsat.2015.09.006

Prince, M., Patel, V., Saxena, S., Maj, M., Maselko, J., Phillips, M. R., & Rahman, A. (2007). No health without mental health. *The Lancet, 370*(9590), 859–877. https://doi.org/10.1016/S0140-6736(07)61238-0

Radez, J., Reardon, T., Creswell, C., Lawrence, P. J., Evdoka-Burton, G., & Waite, P. (2021). Why do children and adolescents (not) see and access professional help for their mental health problems? A systematic review of quantitative and qualitative studies. *European Child & Adolescent Psychiatry, 30*, 183–211. https://doi.org/10.1007/s00787-019-01469-4

Reardon, T., Harvey, K., Baranowska, M., O'Brien, D., Smith, L., & Creswell, C. (2017). What do parents perceive are the barriers and facilitators to accessing psychosocial treatment for mental health problems in children and adolescents? A systematic review of qualitative and quantitative studies. *European Child and Adolescent Psychiatry, 26*(6), 623–647. https://doi.org/10.1007/s00787-016-0930-6

Russo, L., Campagna, I., Ferretti, B., Agricola, E., Pandolfi, E., Carloni, E., D'Ambrosio, A., Gesualdo, F., & Tozzi, A. (2017). What drives attitude towards telemedicine among families of pediatric patients? A survey. *BMC Pediatrics, 17*(21), 21. https://doi.org/10.1186/s12887-016-0756-x

Sayal, K., Tischler, V., Coope, C., Robotham, S., Ashworth, M., Day, C., Tylee, A., & Simonoff, E. (2010). Parental help-seeking in primary care for child and adolescent mental health concerns: Qualitative study. *British Journal of Psychiatry, 197*(6), 476–481. https://doi.org/10.1192/bjp.bp.110.081448

Schwean, V., & Rodger, S. (2013). Children first: it's time to change! Mental health promotion, prevention, and treatment informed by public health, and resiliency approaches. *Canadian Journal of School Psychology, 28*(1), 136–166. https://doi.org/10.1177/0829573513475773

Spaulding, R., Cain, S., & Sonnenschein, K. (2011). Urban telepsychiatry: Uncommon service for a common need. *Child and Adolescent Psychiatric Clinics of North America, 20*(1), 29–39. https://doi.org/10.1016/j.chc.2010.08.010

Sterling, S., Weisner, C., Hinman, A., & Parthasarathy, S. (2010). Access to treatment for adolescents with substance use and co-occurring disorders: Challenges and opportunities. *Journal of the American Academy of Child and Adolescent Psychiatry, 49*(7), 637–646. https://doi.org/10.1016/j.jaac.2010.03.019

Substance Abuse and Mental Health Services Administration (SAMHSA). (n.d.). *Behavioral health integration.* Retrieved from https://www.samhsa.gov/sites/default/files/samhsa-behavioral-health-integration.pdf. Accessed 10 Mar 2024.

Truss, K., Siling, J. L., Phillips, L., Eastwood, O., & Bendall, S. (2023). Barriers to young people seeking help for trauma: A qualitative analysis of internet forums. *Psychological Trauma, 15*(Suppl 1), S163–S171. https://doi.org/10.1037/tra0001344

Watson, A. C., Kelly, B. L., & Vidalon, T. M. (2009). Examining the meaning attached to mental illness and mental health services among justice system-involved youth and their parents. *Qualitative Health Research, 19*(8), 1087–1099. https://doi.org/10.1177/2F1049732309341202

Whaibeh, E., Mahmoud, H., & Naal, H. (2020). Telemental health in the context of a pandemic: The COVID-19 experience. *Current Treatment Options in Psychiatry, 7*(2), 198–202. https://doi.org/10.1007/s40501-020-00210-2

World Health Organization (WHO). (2004). *Promoting mental Health: Concepts, emerging evidence, practice* (Summary report). World Health Organization.

World Health Organization (WHO). (2005). Mental Health: Facing the challenges, building solutions. In *Report from the WHO European ministerial conference*. WHO Regional Office for Europe.

World Health Organization (WHO). (2013). *Mental Health action plan 2013–2020*. World Health Organization. Retrieved from https://apps.who.int/iris/bitstream/handle/10665/89966/9789241506021_eng.pdf?sequence=1. Accessed 10 May 2024

Yoon, Y., Eisenstadt, M., Lereya, S. T., & Deighton, J. (2022). Gender difference in the change of adolescents' mental health and subjective wellbeing trajectories. *European Child & Adolescent Psychiatry, 32*, 1569–1578. https://doi.org/10.1007/2Fs00787-022-01961-4

Zahner, G., Pawelkiewicz, W., DeFrancesco, J. J., & Adnopoz, J. (1992). Children's mental health service needs and utilization patterns in an urban community: An epidemiological assessment. *Journal of the American Academy of Child and Adolescent Psychiatry, 31*(5), 951–960. https://doi.org/10.1097/00004583-199209000-00025

Chapter 10
Lessons, Part III: Public Mental Health Screening for Adolescents

Arthur Maerlender

From a public health perspective, implementing approaches to prevention requires identification of individuals at risk for the specific problem. This is typically addressed through mass screening to identify and monitor those at risk. Typically, those who are at highest risk may be more thoroughly evaluated for potential treatment should they meet clinical criteria.

10.1 Risk Management and Psychometric Adequacy

A systematic process of organizing, forecasting, and evaluating information and identification of procedures to avoid or minimize the potential impact can support risk management. The five steps to identify, analyze, evaluate or rank, monitor, review, and avoid risk play an important role in the process of risk management.

Mental health screening typically employs strategies for identifying behaviors and symptoms that are known to be prodromes of dysfunction and risks of mental illness. This is based on the assumption that mental health is the absence of mental illness. However, it is also possible to screen for the strengths and resources that are necessary for well-being that assumes an absence of mental illness. The choice of the specific screening tool should be based on its psychometrically derived diagnostic/identification utility.

Psychometric adequacy is a must as not all screening tools have been validated to accurately screen certain populations of children and adolescents (e.g., refugee children and adolescents, ethnically diverse groups). Before selecting a tool, schools

A. Maerlender (✉)
Department of Psychology, Saint Anselm College, Manchester, NH, USA

Center for Brain, Biology and Behavior, University of Nebraska – Lincoln, Lincoln, NE, USA
e-mail: amaerlender@anselm.edu; amaerlender2@unl.edu

P. G. Bray, A. Maerlender (eds.), *Adolescent Public Mental Health*,
https://doi.org/10.1007/978-3-031-68294-0_10

	Actually at risk	Actually not at risk	
Poor performance on screening	a) Those screened as 'at risk' and DO have condition (True Positive)	b) Those screened as 'at risk' and DO NOT have condition (False Positive)	Sensitivity = a/(a+b)
Adequate (good) performance on screening	c) Those screened as 'not at risk' and DO have condition (False Negative)	d) Those screened as 'not at risk' and DO NOT have the condition (True Negative)	Specificity = d/(c+d)
	PPV = a/(a+c)	NPV = d/(b+d)	

Fig. 10.1 Signal detection for screening decisions. Note: PPV = positive predictive value; NPV = negative predictive value

should investigate whether it has been studied and found to be effective with the population they intend to screen (Gadeberg & Norredam, 2015; Gadeberg et al., 2017; Glover & Albers, 2007; NCSMH, 2023).

Psychometric adequacy includes being appropriate for age. The method of reporting must reflect the population's self-awareness and may need to rely on confederates to report (e.g., self, parent, or teacher). Younger children typically do not have adequate self-insight for self-report, and thus in these instances, parent or teacher report is more effective (Humphrey & Wigelsworth, 2016).

Thus, a decision to implement screening rests on the purpose of the screening. An important consideration is the "pretest probability" of the disease, disorder, or condition to be prevented. In high prevalence conditions, the goal of screening is typically to rule cases in, while in low prevalence conditions, the goal is often to rule cases out (Bartol, 2015). However, a perfect screening tool has sensitivity and specificity both above 80%. The other metric is a classification of predictive power: that is, the proportion of those identified who truly have the disorder (positive predictive power or PPV) compared to those not identified who truly do not have the disorder (negative predictive power or NPV). These metrics are established in the development process through use of signal detection theory (Shreffler & Huecker, 2023). Figure 10.1 presents a graphical representation of signal detection inputs and outcomes.

10.2 The Youth Risk Behavior Survey

For USA youth in ages 9–12, the CDC administers the Youth Risk Behavior Survey (YRBS) every other year (Box 10.1). The YRBS primarily focuses on assessing behaviors that contribute to the leading causes of death, disability, and social problems among youth and adults. It covers a wide range of health-related behaviors such as substance use, sexual behaviors, violence, and mental health. While the survey may include questions related to mental health, such as depression and suicidal ideation, it typically does not delve extensively into broader aspects of well-being beyond those related to risky behaviors (CDC, n.d.).

The stated purposes of administering the YRBS are to

- Determine how often unhealthy behaviors occur.
- Assess whether unhealthy behaviors increase, decrease, or stay the same over time.
- Provide data at the national, state, territorial and freely associated state, tribal, and local levels.
- Provide data comparing different groups of adolescents.
- Monitor progress toward achieving the Healthy People objectives and other program goals.

The YRBS is a highly regarded survey that is administered to millions of youth and has provided important data; however, its age range overlaps only slightly with adolescence including age 12 as the upper limit. During the pandemic, the CDC implemented the Adolescent Behaviors and Experiences Survey in public high schools to obtain a School Health Profile that covers ages 14–18.

These profiles monitor the status of health education content, physical activity, bullying and sexual harassment, tobacco use and nutrition, school-based health and mental health services, school health coordination, and family and community engagement.

Box 10.1: CDC Youth Risk Behavior System (YRBS)

Ages 9–12

The surveys are administered every other year.

Typically takes 30–45 min

- Measures health-related behaviors and experiences that can lead to death and disability among youth and adults.
- Results help monitor health trends, identify emerging issues, and plan and evaluate programs that can help improve adolescent health.
- Includes high school students from both private and public schools within the USA.
- Surveys conducted by departments of health and education at the state, tribal, territorial, or local levels of their respective public high school students.

Information about

- *Student demographics*: sex, sexual identity, race and ethnicity, and grade.
- *Youth health behaviors and conditions*: sexual, injury and violence, bullying, diet and physical activity, obesity, and mental health, including suicide.

(continued)

Box 10.1 (continued)

- *Substance use behaviors*: electronic vapor product and tobacco product use, alcohol use, and other drug use.
- *Student experiences*: parental monitoring, school connectedness, unstable housing, and exposure to community violence.

Source: CDC (n.d.)

These are important steps and have been shown to be well-received and effective (CDC; also see Li et al., 2022; Szucs et al., 2022). However, these programs are designed to inform policy that would support programmatic efforts, not serve those programs directly. There appears to be no attempt to directly screen for individual mental health or well-being profiles that could provide data for direct intervention.

On the other hand, the multitiered system of supports (MTSS) is a more granular approach specifically designed to inform more specific interventions, albeit at a group level (see earlier chapters for more description about MTSS). Leveraging the success of the YRBS to interface with MTSS programming in schools (e.g., with social emotional learning) would seem a reasonable collaboration across these sectors. However, more attention to resilience and well-being would be welcome.

10.3 Weighing Benefits and Costs of Screening

Screening is very much at the heart of a public health approach. Yet screening for mental health risks is itself somewhat controversial. Clinical screening tools are imprecise and intended to limit false negative findings while accepting false positives on the assumption that individuals may screen positive for many nonclinical reasons and can be weeded out later.

To screen for mental health in schools or not? There are strong opinions on both sides of the issue that are explicated by the Center for Mental Health in Schools at UCLA (2021).

The Center for Mental Health in Schools notes that advocates for whole school screening of mental health see an advantage of early identification of problems before they become debilitating. Such identification should improve student success and reduce costs. Further using schools to support public health programs provides easier access than referral to community programs.

On the other hand, opponents raise cost concerns as well as privacy concerns. Many feel that mental health is a personal matter and will violate rights to privacy, consent, and parental control, despite evidence of the social effects. There are also concerns that by looking for problems, they will be found and resources for care are already too limited. There are also concerns regarding the "false-positive" problem: that is, the inappropriate overidentification of subgroups such as some ethnic groups and boys with externalizing problems and girls with internalizing problems. Relatedly, other arguments are posited regarding insufficient follow-up assessment resources to correct for false-positive identifications.

An important specific consideration is the retraumatization from life-threatening incidents. Screening can help inform how schools should interact with youth in ways that prevent retraumatization of students who report distressing experiences (Overstreet & Chafouleass, 2016). Screening that asks students to describe distressing experiences in detail (e.g., events that were traumatizing) may also generate negative emotions or impacts. Schools should have supports in place to manage and minimize those impacts. For instance, it is important that the screening procedure maximizes student privacy, that there is a school counselor available for students before or after screening, that staff are trained on how to administer tools in a sensitive way, and that students feel safe and grounded when they leave the screening (SAMHSA, 2014).

Further, scarce school time and resources would take from matters not directly related to teaching. Others point to the lack of enough competent school personnel to plan, implement, and evaluate large-scale screening.

Before schools undertake screening, they should have effective connections to the resources necessary to address the student needs that the screening identifies. Such connections might take the form of in-house staffing, partnerships with school- and community-based mental health providers, and virtual (e.g., tele-mental health apps) supports that students and their families can readily access (Siceloff et al., 2017).

Often assumed, the personnel must have knowledge about the tool and understand principles of test administration. On more than one occasion, this author has observed teachers inadvertently "teaching" the test while testing. Competence in test administration is required, as well as maintaining fidelity to the prescribed procedures and instructions. Test reliability is threatened when these conditions are not met.

These are important considerations to be balanced against the increasing social, emotional, and financial costs of adolescent mental illness and despair.

Yet some indirect benefits are also noted such as reducing the stigma around asking youth about mental health within the school setting, enhancing students' sense of empowerment and self-esteem, providing valuable cohort-level information, and learning to adapt to varied perspectives on mental health from youth and families across cultural groups (SAMHSA, 2019).

The reality is that approximately 20% of students show signs and symptoms of a mental health disorder in a given year. Thus, mental health screening can be seen as a proactive approach to gathering valuable information for planning and implementing prevention and early intervention strategies for the other 80% before problems develop or worsen.

As noted, population screening for mental health concerns has been legitimately criticized. Indeed, even population-based screening for epidemic diseases is controversial. In the mental health domain, the criticisms can be serious and legitimate.

Privacy, data security and misuse, improper application and use, and retraumatization are very real problems. Therefore, systems that invoke such screening must be well designed and managed by staff with appropriate expertise in order to assure safe and effective implementation and use (Finkelhor, 2017).

The scope of screening is also important. Universal school mental health screening has been defined as the use of a systematic tool or process to identify both the *strengths* and *needs* of all students. In practice, school-based screening typically only focuses on identifying the risks for or the presence of mental health distress (National Center for School Mental Health, 2023). Collecting data on both mental ill-health and positive mental health at the population level would yield a more complete picture of mental health (Humphrey & Wigelsworth, 2016; OECD, 2023; Suldo & Shaffer, 2008).

Unfortunately, research on the effectiveness of trauma screening in schools and the availability of brief and effective universal screening tools for trauma is accumulating but is still fairly limited (Eklund et al., 2018). Depending on which student needs they are seeking to assess, school leaders may want to consider whether the school is the most effective setting for screening.

10.4 Mental Health or Well-Being?

Particularly at the population level, some aspects of mental health are more frequently captured than others, and there is need for better cross-country harmonizing measures. For instance, screening tools capturing symptoms of depression are more commonly used than those for anxiety. Some countries do capture anxiety, but in nonstandardized ways. Further, affect data are more commonly collected than eudaimonic[1] data, while globally, Organization for Economic Co-operation and Development (OECD) countries are not aligned in the tools used to collect data on positive mental health beyond life satisfaction.

VanderWeele makes the case that if human flourishing is important for "societal good," and connections to family, work, education, and spiritual activity are determinants of flourishing, then "broad human flourishing outcome measures, rather than just specific disease outcomes …should be incorporated into more designs so as to better understand the causes and determinants of, and interventions to promote, human flourishing" (VanderWeele, 2017, p. 8153).

The discipline of positive psychology has proposed various measures of subjective well-being. Typically these measures attempt to assess the constructs of happiness as a positive affective state (sometimes referred to as "hedonic happiness") or overall life satisfaction ("evaluative happiness"). The literature and evidence suggest several different domains, each with their own evaluative tools. There is general

[1] Eudaemonia or eudemonia is the sense of meaning and purpose in life. It is a Greek word for the state or condition of "good spirit," commonly translated as "happiness" or "well-being."

agreement that those domains are (1) happiness and life satisfaction, (2) physical and mental health, (3) meaning and purpose, (4) character and virtue, (5) close social relationship, and (6) financial and material stability. He proposes a 12-item measure called "Flourish" (VanderWeele, 2017).

The OECD report suggests adding four specific tools in relevant population surveys to build a small set of more internationally harmonized population mental health indicators (OECD, 2023).

1. Mental ill-health—priority recommendation: The Patient Health Questionnaire-4 (PHQ-4) could be included in more frequent surveys, alongside the regular collection of the PHQ-8 or PHQ-9 in health surveys. It covers symptoms of both depression and anxiety with only four questions each.
2. Positive mental health—recommendation: Based on trends in country measurement practice, either the Well-Being Index (WHO-5) or the short-form Warwick-Edinburgh Mental Well-Being Scale (SWEMWBS) could be used to measure affective and eudaemonic aspects of positive mental health in a comparative way.
3. General mental health status—recommendation: Similar to questions that ask respondents to rate their physical health, a single question on general mental health status could be included in a range of surveys across a country's broader data infrastructure system. The following framing has been adopted by at least three OECD countries: "In general, how is your mental health? Excellent/Very good/Good/Fair/Poor."

A benefit of screening for well-being is that it does not carry the stigmatizing effect of screening for mental health/illness and gives a proactive message. Additionally, well-being infers influence of the social determinants of health.

10.5 Screening, Equity, and Bias

Further, the approach to screening must be equitable as experiences of racism and the unequal effects on education and mental health due to social determinants of health suggest a need to consider context and experience in order to avoid oppressive practices (Shim et al., 2014). Moore et al. (2023, p. 57) note that there is an important shift with equity-focused mental health screening:

> Equity-focused mental health screening requires a shift from individual- and deficit-focused approaches to systems- and holistic-focused approaches that (a) identify strengths and stressors among individuals, groups, and communities (b) dismantle structural forms of oppression; and (c) promote positive mental health outcomes for minoritized youth.

Ulie-Wells et al. (2020) argue that equitable school-based mental health screening must consider changing the schools, in addition to changing at-risk students. Grounded in critical theoretical frameworks, the recently developed Critical School Mental Health Praxis model can guide decision-making at the intersection of educational equity and mental health in schools (Danelski, 2022; Ulie-Wells et al., 2020).

Prior to engaging in universal mental health screening, several considerations regarding equity are recommended. While most of these have been previously discussed, taken as whole, they provide a useful overview. The process is iterative and interrelated. These considerations include (a) reflecting on the process of systemic change; (b) identifying a team; (c) engaging in ecological assessment; (d) engaging in resource mapping; (e) forming school, family, and community partnerships; (f) clarifying goals and objectives; and (g) selecting an appropriate, technically adequate, and usable tool (Ulie-Wells et al., 2020).

System change is considered a crucial first step in providing equitable mental health screening in schools. A critical question to answer is: "What mental health disparities are most prominent within our school community and most detrimental to students' well-being and social/academic success?" (Sullivan et al., 2015). This often requires analysis of existing records, further data collection, and data disaggregation to get at student group membership (e.g., race and ethnicity, English language proficiency, socioeconomic status, gender identity, sexual orientation). Brown Griffin et al. recommend accounting for students' intersectional identities in the process of data disaggregation (Griffin et al., 2020). Note that focusing on and relying on stereotypes can create disproportionate responses in grading and discipline, for example (Harris, 2022).

Another important query challenges schools to consider ways in which school policies and school climate contribute to both mental health and well-being and prompting administrators to change policies, practices, and procedures before treating (changing) students (Sullivan et al., 2015).

Finally, teachers, students, administrators, and parents should consider what equitable mental health looks like in their particular building. The vision and goals should be specific to the local context and take into consideration the uniqueness and history of the school and community (Sullivan et al., 2015).

Once screening has been conducted, the knowledge gained from the screening must be used to inform equity-explicit practices and may be used to guide policy decisions at local levels. These equity considerations help to connect screening data to specific interventions, including (a) interpreting data to guide follow-up, (b) prioritizing systems-level change, (c) implementing intentional universal (Tier 1) intervention, and (d) engaging in equitable decision-making for Tiers 2 and 3 (Moore et al., 2023).

Although universal mental health screening in schools has potential drawbacks, the benefits would appear to outweigh those risks. Schools are a keystone of a community and it is where adolescents spend a majority of their time. Thus, the schools are the ideal venue for addressing this mental health crisis and supporting this cohort as they move to adulthood. Further, the MTSS approach to structuring student learning creates continuous performance feedback that enables ongoing *behavioral* monitoring at a group level. While individuals may still "fall through the cracks," it is less likely.

From a public health perspective, effective screening can assist schools and communities in understanding the magnitude of risks, thus informing better implementation of prevention and promotion strategies that are at the heart of the public health mission. Expanding the scope of preventative screening and promotion to include well-being and resilience creates a structure for positive education and thus balances the focus on deficits. Further, by focusing on equitable development and implementation, benefits accrue to the entire community. But this endeavor cannot be taken lightly. It should be thought out and prepared in advance of implementation. The Moore et al. (2023) *Roadmap* paper should be required reading for those embarking on this process.

Competing Interests *The author has no conflicts of interest to declare that are relevant to the content of this chapter.*

References

Bartol, T. (2015). Thoughtful use of diagnostic testing: Making practical sense of sensitivity, specificity, and predictive value. *The Nurse Practitioner, 40*(8), 10–12. https://doi.org/10.1097/01.NPR.0000470366.64804.35

CDC (Centers for Disease Control and Prevention). (n.d.). *The youth risk behavior surveillance survey*. https://www.cdc.gov/healthyyouth/data/yrbs/index.htm. Retrieved 20 April, 2024.

Center for Mental Health in Schools at UCLA. (2021). *Screening for mental health problems in school*. https://www.smhp.psych.ucla.edu/pdfdocs/policyissues/mhscreeningissues.pdf. Retrieved 21 Dec. 2023. This brief provides responses and documentation for the following: How appropriate is large-scale screening for mental health problems? Will the costs of large-scale mental health screening programs outweigh the benefits? Are schools an appropriate venue for large-scale screening of mental health problems?

Danelski, D. (2022, December 21). *Analysis calls for bias-free mental health screenings to uplift students and neighborhoods*. Medical Xpress. Retrieved December 21, 2023, from https://medicalxpress.com/news/2022-12-analysis-bias-free-mental-health-screenings.html

Eklund, K., Rossen, E., Koriakin, T., Chafouleas, S.M., Resnick, C. (2018). A systematic review of trauma screening measures for children and adolescents. *School Psychology Quarterly, 33*(1), 30–43. https://doi.org/10.1037/spq0000244. PMID: 29629787.

Finkelhor, D. (2017). Screening for adverse childhood experiences (ACEs): Cautions and suggestions. *Child Abuse and Neglect, 85*, 174–179. https://doi.org/10.1016/j.chiabu.2017.07.016

Gadeberg, A., & Norredam, M. (2015). Urgent need for validated trauma and mental health screening tools for refugee children and youth. *European Child and Adolescent Psychiatry, 25*(8), 929–931. https://doi.org/10.1007/s00787-016-0837-2

Gadeberg, A., Montgomery, E., Frederiksen, H., & Norredam, M. (2017). Assessing trauma and mental health in refugee children and youth: A systematic review of validated screening and measurement tools. *European Journal of Public Health, 27*(3), 439–446. https://doi.org/10.1093/eurpub/ckx034

Glover, T. A., & Albers, C. A. (2007). Considerations for evaluating universal screening assessments. *Journal of School Psychology, 45*(2), 117–135. https://doi.org/10.1016/j.jsp.2006.05.005

Griffin, C., Metzger, I., Halliday-Boykins, C. A., & Salazar, C. A. (2020). Racial fairness, school engagement, and discipline outcomes in African American high school students: The important role of gender. *School Psychology Review, 49*(3), 222–238. https://doi.org/10.1080/2372966X.2020.1726810

Harris, J. N. (2022). When they *don't* see us: Using intersectionality to examine Black girls' discipline experiences. In S. Proctor & D. Rivera (Eds.), *Critical theories for school psychology and counseling: A foundation for equity and inclusion in school-based practice* (pp. 83–100). Routledge.

Humphrey, N., & Wigelsworth, M. (2016). Making the case for universal school-based mental health screening. *Emotional and Behavioural Difficulties, 21*(1), 22–42. https://doi.org/10.1080/13632752.2015.1120051

Li, J., Timpe, Z., Suarez, N. A., Phillips, E., Kaczkowski, W., Cooper, A. C., Dittus, P. J., Robin, L., Barrios, L. C., & Ethier, K. A. (2022). Dosage in implementation of an effective school-based health program impacts youth health risk behaviors and experiences. *The Journal of Adolescent Health, 71*(3), 334–343. https://doi.org/10.1016/j.jadohealth.2022.04.009

Moore, S., Long, A. C. J., Coyle, S., Cooper, J. M., Mayworm, A. M., Amirazizi, S., Edyburn, K. L., Pannozzo, P., Choe, C., Miller, F. G., Eklund, K., Bohnenkamp, J., Whitcomb, S., Raines, T. C., & Dowdy, E. (2023). A roadmap to equitable school mental health screening. *Journal of School Psychology, 96*, 57–74.

National Center for School Mental Health (NCSMH). (2023). *School mental health quality guide: Screening*. NCSMH, University of Maryland School of Medicine. https://www.schoolmentalhealth.org/media/som/microsites/ncsmh/documents/quality-guides-2023/Screening-Quality-Guide-2023.pdf

OECD: Organisation for Economic Co-operation and Development. (2023). *Measuring population mental health*. OECD Publishing. www.oecd-ilibrary.org/content/publication/5171eef8-en

Overstreet, S., & Chafouleas, S. (2016). Trauma-informed schools: Introduction to the special issue. *School Mental Health, 8*(1), 1–6. https://link.springer.com/article/10.1007/s12310-016-9184-1#CR14

SAMHSA (Substance Abuse and Mental Health Services Administration). (2014). Screening and assessment. In *Trauma informed care in behavioral health services* (Treatment improvement protocol series, No. 57 (ch. 4)). Center for Substance Abuse Treatment. https://www.ncbi.nlm.nih.gov/books/NBK207188/

SAMHSA (Substance Abuse and Mental Health Services Administration). (2019). *Ready, set, go, review: Screening for behavioral health risk in schools*. Office of the Chief Medical Officer, Substance Abuse and Mental Health Services Administration. https://www.samhsa.gov/sites/default/files/ready-set-go-review-mh-screening-schools.pdf

Shim, R., Koplan, R. C., Langheim, F. J. P., Manseau, M. W., Powers, R. A., & Compton, M. T. (2014). The social determinants of mental health: An overview and call to action. *Psychiatric Annals, 44*(1), 22–26. https://doi.org/10.3928/00485713-20140108-04

Shreffler, J. & Huecker, M. (2023, March 6). *Diagnostic testing accuracy: Sensitivity, specificity, predictive values and likelihood ratios*. StatPearls (Internet). https://www.ncbi.nlm.nih.gov/books/NBK557491/. Retrieved 10 May 2024

Siceloff, R., Bradley, J., & Flory, K. (2017). Universal behavioral/emotional health screening in schools: Overview and feasibility. *Report on Emotional and Behavioral Disorders in Youth, 17*(2), 32–38. https://www.ncbi.nlm.nih.gov/pmc/articles/PMC6350819/

Suldo, S. M., & Shaffer, E. J. (2008). Looking beyond psychopathology: The dual-factor model of mental health in youth. *School Psychology Review, 37*(1), 52–68.

Sullivan, A. L., Artiles, A. J., & Hernandez-Saca, D. J. (2015). Addressing special education inequity through systemic change: Contributions of ecologically based organizational consultation. *Journal of Educational and Psychological Consultation, 25*(2–3), 129–147. https://doi.org/10.1080/10474412.2014.929969

Szucs, L. E., Harper, C. R., Andrzejewski, J., Barrios, L. C., Robin, L., & Hunt, P. (2022). Overwhelming support for sexual health education in U.S. schools: A meta-analysis of 23 surveys conducted between 2000 and 2016. *The Journal of Adolescent Health, 70*(4), 598–606. https://doi.org/10.1016/j.jadohealth.2021.05.016

Ulie-Wells, J., Bruna, K. R., & Romo, C. (2020). Critical school mental health praxis (CrSMHP): A framework for change. In C. Clauss-Ehlers, A. Sood, & M. Weist (Eds.), *Social justice for children and young people: International perspectives* (pp. 175–193). Cambridge University Press. https://doi.org/10.1017/9781108551830.012

VanderWeele, T. (2017). On the promotion of human flourishing. *Proceedings of the National Academy of Sciences, 114*(31), 8148–8156. https://doi.org/10.1073/pnas.1702996114PERSPECTIVE

Chapter 11
Taking Action with the Adolescent Public Mental Health Model

Arthur Maerlender and Patricia Gail Bray

11.1 Introduction

Globally many public health programs have been developed and implemented to address mental illness and its prevention, with specific attention to schools. The call for better integration of mental health services into medical care clinics has also been an important development. Some schools have had mental health clinics within their walls for many years. Middle and high schools are where adolescents spend most of their time, so focusing on service delivery in association with these educational institutions seems prudent. The thesis throughout this volume asserts that sometimes solution-driven, stand-alone *programs* are not sufficient to improve the broken adolescent mental health system. A question then is, what actions are necessary to make a transformative systems change with adolescent mental health?

In their worksheet on best practices, the National Center for Safe, Supportive Learning (NCSSF) notes that interest and investment in school mental health has grown in the past two decades. Yet identifying effective programs for integrating mental health and behavioral health services in schools is in need of research and

Supplementary Information The online version contains supplementary material available at https://doi.org/10.1007/978-3-031-68294-0_11.

A. Maerlender (✉)
Department of Psychology, Saint Anselm College, Manchester, NH, USA

Center for Brain, Biology and Behavior, University of Nebraska – Lincoln, Lincoln, NE, USA
e-mail: amaerlender@anselm.edu; amaerlender2@unl.edu

P. G. Bray
Department of Management, Policy and Community Health, UTHealth Houston School of Public Health, The University of Texas Health Science Center (UTHealth) at Houston, Houston, TX, USA

P. G. Bray, A. Maerlender (eds.), *Adolescent Public Mental Health*,
https://doi.org/10.1007/978-3-031-68294-0_11

guidance to overcome difficulties in resourcing and implementing the changes (NCSSF, n.d.; also see Atkins et al., 2010). Schools in some countries have adapted a public health approach to learning and well-being through the multitiered system of supports. However, schools have also reported difficulties in implementing programs for a variety of reasons: Those include but are not limited to staff buy-in, limited school personnel time and resources, school accountability emphasizing academic to the exclusion of social-emotional outcomes, and limited parent involvement (Forman et al., 2009; Langley et al., 2010).

Doing nothing will maintain or increase the impact of poor adolescent mental health and is not cost-effective, given the scope of the crisis. While many potential solutions are in existence, albeit in a piecemeal, distributed manner, addressing the barriers to change requires a clear commitment to create a critical mass of action.

11.2 What Is the Cost of Action? What Is the Cost of Inaction?

Le et al. (2021) reviewed 65 studies of the cost-effectiveness of mental health promotion and prevention interventions from 2008 to 2020. Utilizing a definition of mental health that focuses on well-being, the authors noted that promoting positive mental health and well-being in order to prevent mental illness has become a priority across many sectors and jurisdictions (See also, Galderisi et al., 2015; World Health Organization, 2004). Study targets ranged from suicide prevention to promoting mental health to universal employee wellness programs.

For children and adolescents under 18 years, 23 studies evaluated the cost-effectiveness of 33 active interventions for mental health prevention and promotion versus groups with no intervention or a wait list control. The majority of studies were from high-income countries (the USA, Australia, Sweden, the UK, the Netherlands) and one multinational study. The authors noted that, given the known effects of social determinants of (mental) health, the limited evidence from low- and middle-income countries misses a critical piece of the problem.

The considerable evidence of the links between social determinants and mental health outcomes indicates that multilevel interventions aimed at eliminating systemic social inequalities are crucial (Alegría et al., 2018; World Health Organization, 2014). These include, for example, access to educational and employment opportunities, healthy food, secure housing, and safe neighborhoods (Alegría et al., 2018; World Health Organization, 2014).

Importantly, a framework for analysis of the social determinants of health of child well-being designed by Bell et al. (2013, pp. 13–14)[1] in middle- and lower-income countries incorporated the individual, family, systems (e.g., health,

[1] The framework was adapted from the WHO European review of social determinants of health and the health divide (Marmot et al., 2012).

education), societal (e.g., social norms), and macro (e.g., political, economic) levels. Their argument stated that since the culmination of all the various factors affects children's mental health outcomes, the research approach can be expanded to include ways to target these factors to improve children's outcomes.

In the USA, attaining population levels of well-being is hampered by current motivational (incentive) structures that focus on extrinsic reinforcement. Healthcare systems that are solely driven by profit motives are not conducive to the types of cooperative, multisystem, organizational behaviors required. For acute illness care, industry profit motives are inherently extrinsic and, as such, fuel competitive corporate goals contrary to individual needs. Yet despite the evidence, cost savings from mental illness prevention and mental health wellness promotion are often too distant for quarterly management and thus not fully embraced.

11.2.1 Adolescent Research and Practice

While clinical science and practice have known for over a century that there are important developmental markers that occur during adolescence that can have lifelong effects, the attempts at addressing adolescents as a unique group have been fragmented and disjointed. One factor has been the apparent disconnect between conditions of mental illness and mental health, physical illness and physical health, and the interrelationships of well-being and social determinants of health.

Although individuals need effective access to illness care, incorporating preventative approaches that are integrated into the illness-care system will reduce costs and improve outcomes. Research points to the importance of early detection of risk factors and incipient disease through screening as effective tools in this regard. While screening carries its own concerns (e.g., misuse of data and privacy), a balance must be struck with guardrails for protection of individuals and groups. For children and adolescents, a review on the cost-effectiveness of mental health prevention and promotion interventions found that screening and psychological intervention at school were the most cost-effective for prevention of mental disorders (Le et al., 2021). Supporting mental and physical health is far more efficient and cost-effective than treating illness.

11.2.2 Adolescent Public Mental Health

The argument put forth here is that an adolescent public mental health system of prevention and care is required—a system that links prevention, clinical mental healthcare, schools, and communities. Schools are a part of a broader community of stakeholders in sustainable well-being, which includes parents, neighbors, businesses, local health departments, and healthcare providers. Adolescents are the proverbial canaries in the coal mine as they grow into their adult form, making a wraparound approach focused on health a crucial population support.

A primary mandate from Kania and Kramer (2011) is that community action requires a commitment from all of these stakeholders—a commitment that is reified and reinforced continually. Business leaders speak of total quality improvement (TQI); a proven method of TQI is the collective impact (CI) approach (Kania & Kramer, 2011). This governance structure provides ongoing commitment, support, and monitoring of activities in real time, across sectors, that fosters and guides progress while making changes as needed.

11.3 How Would Communities Have to Change?

Communities must first accept that their adolescent population is a potential productive resource and key to population stability. They are the community's future and the promise, or their pitfall.

Communities have the ability to adopt a system-level approach to solving problems of this nature. The community's task is to, first, make adolescent public mental health a priority. Second, they would need to get commitments from public health, healthcare and mental health leaders, and education leaders to make a commitment to change. Proven tools such as collective impact are readily available but require direct involvement and commitment of the sector leaders (see below). For instance, in the USA, this might include the director of community mental health, the superintendent of schools, CEOs of funding organizations, and participating healthcare providers. Further, these leaders must reaffirm their commitments on a regular basis, based on progress reports and feedback from the ground-level managers and staff. Such regular, ongoing top-level management with direct connection to bottom-level activity has been shown to maintain positive outcomes while supporting necessary adaptations and changes.

Third, this process should develop as a sustainable, ongoing governance function until population well-being is an established value in the community.

11.4 How Would Public Health Have to Change?

Public health has shown its responsiveness most recently through the COVID-19 pandemic. It is the system ideally suited to colead the efforts that are called for. Public health professionals are skilled at health promotion and prevention, intervention design, education and awareness, community engagement, equity, and the social determinants of health.

First and foremost, a change in language is needed. "Health" can no longer be viewed as either physical health *or* mental health. "Health" is both, as there cannot be one without the other. The term "well-being" perhaps best captures the essence of both. What this means is that prevention of physical and mental illness should focus on supporting health and well-being. Public health has experience in methods of disease prevention and health promotion. That can and should include school-based health enhancing programs.

Leading the way in the development and implementation of effective, nonintrusive approaches to population-level screening with privacy protections in place would be invaluable. Active supports to address inequities in the social determinants of "health" will be needed, and, as taxpayer funded organizations, local public health departments have access to leaders and leverage, as do conventional healthcare providers.

11.5 How Would Mental Health Have to Change?

A Mental Health State of the World Report released in March 2024 by the Global Mind Project ranks the USA 29th out of 71 countries (Global Mind Project, 2024). As implied above, mental health services need to be more integrated into physical healthcare, as well as non-health related services including education. This realization has increased since COVID-19, which is a positive sign. The limiting step in this process is the current fragmentation of the healthcare system into separate mental and physical health systems of care. A more integrated system of care delivery is imperative, or the USA will continue to be at the bottom of healthcare for developed countries (See Commonwealth Fund, 2023).

Currently in the USA, mental healthcare is focused on treatment of mental illness. Instead of only treatment, positive mental *health* promotion, mental illness prevention, and early intervention need to become part of the "care" system.

Mental health promotion and mental illness prevention identify disorders earlier, rather than later, and could help alleviate the bottleneck regarding access to care. Even in a perfect preventative world, clinical care is needed. The BridgeUp model (discussed in a previous chapter) demonstrated the value of rapid access to care for adolescents when needed. Healthcare leaders have to commit to providing this kind of service, first.

Providing acute care is also important. Many schools now feature on-site clinics and services. As a community member, these clinics could also be open to other community population subsets. Interestingly, as the population shifts, school enrollments are plummeting and well-built school structures are becoming empty. Those investments can be enhanced by creative community usage, such as care clinics.

11.6 How Would Schools Have to Change?

Partnering with public heath for development of school health programs would be an important prevention tool. At the state level, public health departments are familiar and expert in health prevention activities and can target specific populations.

Additionally, another potential partnership could the establishment of a commitment from local health and mental health agencies and providers to collaborate with schools to provide easy and seamless access to crisis care and treatment. While the goal of APMH is prevention and early intervention, the reality is that the crisis is ongoing and even when subsided, individuals need access and care. Immediate access is critical. The BridgeUp program's partnership with a large mental health organization provided access to 63,325 students, and some of the schools had clinics on-site (see Jo Jo's story in a previous chapter).

School-based programs that develop proactive skills are already in place and have been shown to be effective. As mentioned in the earlier School Health chapter, multitiered system of supports (MTSS) for mental wellness and social-emotional learning (SEL) have roots in public health and prevention. Implementation of social and behavioral learning programs such as SEL has been shown to improve school engagement, reduce disciplinary referrals, and improve academic performance while making for more stable and effective educational environments (Durlak et al., 2015).

However, in the social-behavioral realm, screening for the identification of risk can be controversial, even though necessary. Rather than screen for mental health problems, one approach is to screen for well-being. There are observable behavioral indicators that when applied systematically and with high fidelity can serve such a purpose. Indicators of positive mental health such as curiosity, persistence, and self-control can be incorporated into MTSS programming (see Bitsko et al., 2022). The Collaborative for Academic, Social, and Emotional Learning (CASEL-5) competencies could be another approach and includes (1) self-awareness, (2) social awareness, (3) self-management, (4) developing relational skills, and (5) developing decision-making skills (Collaborative for Academic, Social and Emotional Learning, 2021).

Based on their review of the research, NCSSF (n.d.) makes six recommendations (see Box 11.1) to seek funding for implementation of comprehensive, effective, and sustainable approaches for preventing, identifying, and treating mental health in schools, including addressing violence and trauma.

Box 11.1: National Center for Safe, Supportive Learning Environments Best Practices for Implementing School Mental Health Supports

1. Align Programs Across a Continuum of Services
   - Provide MTSS for positive behavior, social-emotional learning, and school climate to reduce the need for mental health services and align with academic programming.
2. Incorporate Youth and Family Voices
   - Obtain student and parent perceptions of needs, including representative parent advisory groups for ongoing communication. Reach out to existing community organizations to provide joint activities.

(continued)

Box 11.1 (continued)

3. Engage Leadership in Implementation Planning and Support
   - Involve leadership across school, district, and state levels in the planning of mental health programming early on with a focus on program linkages. Address school disciplinary policies about interventions and approaches that support student mental health.
4. Build Staff Mental Health Capacity
   - Provide whole-school and district-wide training to promote knowledge of mental health concerns like trauma or depression. Explore opportunities for funding staff professional development time. Include teacher mentoring and coaching utilizing existing resources. Make sure to include staff well-being in the matrix of service.
5. Utilize Data for Continuous Quality Improvement (CQI)
   - Systematically collect relevant data capturing appropriate characteristics (such as demographic information) and inputs such as staff training, interventions, and outcomes, including baseline data. Develop data management support systems with technical assistance when available, ideally with support from someone with dedicated time for these responsibilities (i.e., data specialist). Training in data utilization and reporting is also important.
6. Build School-Community Partnerships[2]
   - Develop programmatic collaborations with evidence-based programs. Develop processes that ensure clear responsibilities and regular two-way communication (e.g., memorandum of understanding), which should be informed by and shared with site leadership. Community partners should be educated about local school cultures, and all partners must be accountable for their commitments.

Source: NCSSF (n.d.)

Finally, moving to a community school model has important attributes that support the well-being of students while adding substantive value to the larger community (Covelli et al., 2022). However, community schools vary in the programs offered and are typically based on local priorities and contexts. However, four "pillars" of community schools are generally observed (Maier et al., 2017).

According to Maier et al. (2017), the first pillar is *integrated student supports*, which attends to the whole child, including academic, social, emotional, physical,

[2] See Coalition for Community Schools, 2020; Covelli et al., 2022 and Purpose Built Communities, 2024. A BridgeUp school was part of a formal purpose built community.

psychological, and moral development. The second pillar, *expanded learning time and opportunities*, provides additional and sufficient resources for applied, meaningful learning and opportunities. The third pillar is *family and community engagement*, which expands the school to serve as a neighborhood hub that helps to build a broader base of community safety and trust. The fourth pillar, *collaborative leadership and practice*, integrates multisector partnerships to strengthen and support teachers with professional learning and learning communities.

The four community school pillars align closely with evidence-based features of good schools, derived from decades of research identifying school characteristics that foster students' intellectual, social, emotional, and physical development (see, e.g., Bryk et al., 2010; Duncan & Murnane, 2014; Hattie, 2008; Purkey & Smith, 1983). These pillars are integrated into the five principles of the APMH model.

Maier et al. (2017) reported 12 findings that qualify the community schools' approach as an evidence-based intervention under ESSA (Every Student Succeeds Act). According to the US Department of Education's Office of Elementary and Secondary Education (2020), the four tiers of evidence-based practices are defined as follows:

- Tier 1 Strong Evidence: Evidence from at least one well-designed and well-implemented experimental study.
- Tier 2 Moderate Evidence: Evidence from at least one well-designed and well-implemented quasi-experimental study.
- Tier 3 Promising Evidence: Evidence from at least one well-designed and well-implemented correlational study with statistical controls for selection bias.
- Tier 4 Demonstrates a Rationale: Rationale is based on high-quality research findings or positive evaluation that such activity, strategy, or intervention is likely to improve student outcomes or other relevant outcomes and includes ongoing efforts to examine the effects of such activity, strategy, or intervention.

Examples of the Maier et al. (2017) findings include reduced absenteeism, improved academic outcomes, and student reports of more positive school climates, which align with the BridgeUp outcomes, reported in an earlier chapter.

11.7 Systems Change Through Collective Impact

Meaningful systems change requires collaboration across sectors (Rittel & Webber, 1973). Defined by Bryson et al. (2006, p. 44) as "partnerships involving government, business, nonprofits and philanthropies, communities, and/or the public as a whole," cross-sector collaboration has long been a strategy for addressing entrenched social problems such as addiction, environmental health justice, and health disparities (Butterfoss & Kegler, 2009; Roussos & Fawcett, 2000). A variety of theories, models, frameworks, and principles for cross-sector collaborations are proposed in the scientific literature as well as through practitioner-oriented organizations and publications (deMontigny et al., 2019). In 2002, Butterfoss and Kegler noted that "the practice of coalition building has outpaced the development of coalition theory" (Butterfoss & Kegler, 2009, p. 161).

Since then, practitioners and researchers have expanded the repertoire of cross-sector collaboration frameworks used to plan, support, and evaluate these entities. Such cross-sector collaborations represent different activities in a community, such as healthcare, education, community residents, and government, allowing each to contribute their unique perspectives, resources, capabilities, and social capital toward a shared vision that could not be achieved by organizations acting within a single sector (Bryson et al., 2006). Such collaborative strategies have been eagerly adopted as a means to improve health through community-based efforts. The community coalition action theory (CCAT) was developed as a comprehensive theory of community coalitions to inform more effective models of successful implementation (Butterfoss & Kegler, 2009).

Collective impact (CI) is a framework for community change efforts designed to focus on shifting systems, policy, and environments. It is based on the assumption that true change requires the cooperation and coordination of multiple community sectors, rather than from the isolated interventions of individual organizations where no single entity has the authority or resources to bring about the necessary change. Kania and Kramer (2011) distinguish "collective impact" from collaboration by agreeing to a set of principles and behaviors. Agreement to align the work around a shared goal is a distinguishing mark of collective impact as compared to collaboration (Collins et al., 2016).

A primary goal of the CI approach is to bring a diverse set of stakeholders together to agree to address a complex social or environmental problem. Engaging different sectors in such an agreement is critical. Their goals are to focus on root causes and to monitor progress toward the solution over time. As Wolff has opined, they must acknowledge the relative failures of cross-sector collaboration to address social justice concerns (Wolff, 2016, p. 4).

A systematic review of peer-reviewed research on CI identified 19 articles about its use in various settings (Ennis & Tofa, 2019). The objective was to understand successful usage of CI in various large social change projects. Overall, the articles supported CI as an important tool for promoting discussions of social change and collaboration. Four themes were identified: a need to define the specific context and boundaries of the project, having the technical skills needed to implement CI, the critical importance of the relationship-building aspect, and the lack of attention to social equity, power, and grassroots engagement.

A systematic review of CI implementation across a broad range of public health issues identified 95 articles that involved cross-sector collaboration to address chronic diseases, cancer prevention, obesity, mental health, and maternal and child health (Calancie et al., 2021). The projects described primarily focused on health promotion, improving health systems, and substance abuse reduction. Less frequently reported topics were about access to healthcare, community health, and specific diseases or health concerns. Although the studies were varied in design and methodology, the review focused on several domains. These domains of interest included the organizational structure and internal processes, the group, available social capital, activities within the collaboration, activities within the broader community, and activities in both the collaboration and in the community. Fifty-seven percent (57%) of the articles were either case studies or reports on "lessons from the field." Twenty-six percent included more than one collaboration offering a cross-sectional analysis, 12% were conceptual papers with no data to report, and only two articles (2%) reported community-level outcomes.

Although some of the CI studies reported positive results, others noted limitations of the model. Importantly, few of the studies reported outcomes, making comparison of effects difficult, while the broad scope of categorical results further complicated comparisons. Still, studies have generally concluded that cross-sector collaboration is needed to address root causes of persistent social problems, including those related to public health.

To the previous point, a systematic scoping review by Panjwani et al. (2023) identified challenges in evaluating implementation and outcomes of 18 CI initiatives that met study criteria. Effective evaluation was a frequent concern, with CI complexity mentioned as an impediment to effective evaluation. Design and implementation of context-specific methods and ongoing reporting of results were recommended. The authors noted that the planning stage was critical for addressing these concerns.

11.8 Addressing Equity in Collective Impact

Why include equity in collective impact? As Kania et al. (2022) note, equity is included since functionally lack of equity is a barrier to cooperative collaboration that in turn requires trust and respect. Centering equity at the heart of systems change work is critically important for gaining a deep understanding of problems and potential solutions and addressing power imbalances that are often at the heart of problems in society. Addressing issues of equity begins with understanding who has been marginalized and why and how they are experiencing marginalization. Once there is an understanding of the who, where, why, and how for the targeted actions, then actions regarding creating policies, practices, and institutions that address current and historical inequities can be taken (Kania et al., 2022).

Addressing historical inequities can be both challenging and liberating. The process confers a sense of trust in the organizations by demonstrating the need to understand the roots of the problem and the willingness to address those roots and not just the current manifestations of the problem.

For example, Kania et al. (2022) relate that in Chattanooga, Tennessee, the CI process led to a realization that there was not a shared lexicon of the meaning of equity by all of the participants in their project. In effect, semantics was at the core of misunderstanding. By coming to terms, the project was able to understand the roots of the problem and "explicitly named and addressed power

Box 11.2: Strategies for Centering Equity

1. Ground the work in data and context, and target solutions.
2. Focus on systems change, in addition to programs and services.
3. Shift power within the collaborative.
4. Listen to and act with community.
5. Build equity leadership and accountability.

Source: Kania et al. (2022)

imbalances that affected communication and relationships among participants" (Kania et al., 2022, p. 40).

Thus, centering equity in a systems-changing CI approach requires rethinking the "supposed facts that define the problem by recognizing that marginalized populations within any community have experiences that are very different from those of many individuals and organizations who work to help them" (Kania et al., 2022, p. 40). This process gets at the heart of language and how conditions and experiences are described and felt. This was the case with the BridgeUp case study and is reflected in the lessons learned chapters.

In synthesizing efforts to address equity in changing systems worldwide, Kania et al. (2022) synthesized five basic strategy principles that, when taken together, form the basis of a comprehensive and integrated approach to centering equity in collective impact (see Box 11.2; Kania et al., 2022, p. 41).

11.9 Taking Action

Drawing on the findings and experience reported here and in earlier chapters, four kinds of recommendations are proposed with the adoption of the adolescent public mental health model. Each of these is separable and could precede adoption of others. However, our experience suggests that they are mutually reinforcing and can ease the way for broader model implementation and greater scale. Taking action includes the following four classes of recommendations:

1. The nature and processes of adolescent assessment
2. School funding, function, and programming
3. The content and direction of research
4. The scope and scale of collaboration

The 24 suggested recommendations appear in Box 11.3.

Box 11.3 Taking Action With the Adolescent Public Mental Health Model

Assessment

1. Adopt a whole child approach: integration of mind/body with mental/physical health to offer and train pediatricians and other mental health clinicians in mental health issues.
2. Train teachers, public health practitioners, primary care physicians, pediatricians, mental health counselors, and psychologists to integrate prevention, and the social determinants of health, with treatment.
3. Include integrated emotional screening with the well-child visit, similar to vision, hearing, and body mass index, including whole child screening for child and adolescent depression, anxiety, ADHD, and suicide in primary care settings.
4. As part of MTSS, school clinical staff should implement standardized mental health screenings for those showing signs or symptoms and may need acute care.
5. Address the problems of categorical diagnoses inherent in the *Diagnostic Statistical Manual* (DSM).
6. Integrate approaches to SDOH and equity through mental health literacy, mental health access for adolescents, and multisector collaboration.

Schools

1. Expand the cognitive and noncognitive teaching in schools (ESSA) so students learn about improving life skills that affect mental health and well-being.
2. Expand all school classes to teach mental health literacy to reinforce healthy relationships, decision-making, and social-emotional intelligence.
3. Foster intrinsic motivation in youth, such as autonomy, mastery, and purpose.
4. Implement the adolescent public mental health model to continue the movement toward SEL integration with MTSS in schools, along with protocols for immediate mental health supports, when needed.
5. Fund nurturing and supportive schools (including start times based on biological realities).
6. Make schools centers of the community with multiple uses that serve everyone.

Research

1. Adopt a social ecological model for all adolescent mental health research.
2. Explore more research with puberty, social brain mapping, and SEL education.

(continued)

Box 11.3 (continued)

3. Include well-being as an outcome of mental health.
4. Address the underlying inequalities and omissions with the social determinants of health.
5. Study effective and efficient ways to increase capacity and access to quality acute care.
6. Create and track evaluation metrics for public mental health interventions.
7. Study how to take evidence-based prevention and social determinants of health interventions to scale, support, and sustain these interventions, and learn what adaptations might be needed for programs designed in high-income countries to be effective in low- and middle-income countries.
8. Develop adolescent population databases including efficacious preventive policies and programs across mental health problems and health outcomes; the structural and intermediate determinants they address; population health real time from the global, national, state, and local screenings; and community surveys that comprehensively measure structural determinants and mental health.

Multisector Collaboration

1. Develop sustainable adolescent public mental health multisector systems.
2. Utilize collective impact to include multi-stakeholder concerns and needs with the adolescent mental health systems.
3. Ensure that policymakers, practitioners, scientists, and the general public are made aware of the health, social benefits and cost savings, and evidence-based preventive interventions in adolescent mental health.
4. Include a combination of effective, multisector preventive policies and programs before and during the second decade of life.

11.10 The Future

This book's themes of prevention of mental illness, inclusion of the social determinants of health, promotion of positive mental health and well-being, multisector and multisystem cooperation, and cost-effective approaches all coalesce to provide a new view with the adolescent public mental health model. This requires a redirection and different foci since "mental ill-health represents the main threat to the health, survival and future potential of young people around the world" (McGorry et al., 2022. p. 61).

Many of these changes are already in place in diverse locations in the USA and around the world and represent macro-level investments in energy and commitment. Still, there are significant barriers that must be overcome in any specific locale. The concepts and strategies of systems change and collective impact offer a viable road map for developing and sustaining adolescent public health programs that are efficient and cost-effective and that will necessarily prepare our future adults with skills and behaviors needed in the mid- to late twenty-first century.

Nothing speaks to the future better than adolescents. The embedded video presents an example of the power of a changed system using the CI approach across multiple sectors in Houston, Texas. Meet Keylen Evans, who was a senior at Ball High School in Galveston, Texas, in 2022 (Video 11.1). He was part of the BridgeUp project during high school. Today Keylen is a rising junior in college, majoring in aerospace engineering.

Competing Interests *The authors have no conflicts of interest to declare that are relevant to the content of this chapter.*

References

Alegría, M., DeMoyer, A., Falgàs Bagué, I., Wang, Y., & Alvarez, K. (2018). Social determinants of mental health: Where we are and where we need to go. *Current Psychiatry Reports, 20*(11), 95. https://doi.org/10.1007/s11920-018-0969-9

Atkins, M. S., Hoagwood, K. E., Kutash, K., & Seidman, E. (2010). Toward the integration of education and mental health in schools. *Administration and Policy in Mental Health, 37*(1–2), 40–47. https://doi.org/10.1007/s10488-010-0299-7

Bell, R., Donkin, A., & Marmot, M. (2013). Tackling structural and social issues to reduce inequities in children's outcomes in low-to middle-income countries. UCL Institute of Health Equity, UNICEF. Retrieved April 15, 2024, from https://www.instituteofhealthequity.org/resources-reports/tackling-structural-and-social-issues-to-reduce-inequities-in-childrens-outcomes-in-low-to-middle-income-countries/tackling-structural-and-social-issues-to-reduce-inequities.pdf

Bitsko, R. H., Claussen, A. H., Lichtstein, J., Black, L. J., Everett Jones, S., Danielson, M. D., Hoenig, J. M., Davis Jack, S. P., Brody, D. J., Gyawali, S., Maenner, M. M., Warner, M., Holland, K. M., Perou, R., Crosby, A. E., Blumberg, S. J., Avenevoli, S., Kaminski, J. W., & Ghandour, R. M. (2022). Surveillance of children's mental health—United States, 2013–2019. *MMWR, 71*(Suppl-2), 1–42.

Bryk, A. S., Sebring, P. B., Allensworth, E., Easton, J. Q., & Luppescu, S. (2010). *Organizing schools for improvement: Lessons from Chicago*. University of Chicago Press.

Bryson, J. M., Crosby, B. C., & Stone, M. M. (2006). The design and implementation of cross-sector collaborations: Propositions from the literature. *Public Administration Review, 66*, 44–55. https://doi.org/10.1111/j.1540-6210.2006.00665.x

Butterfoss, F. D., & Kegler, M. C. (2009). The community coalition action theory (Ch 9). In R. J. DiClemente, R. A. Crosby, & M. C. Kegler (Eds.), *Emerging theories in health promotion practice and research* (2nd ed., pp. 237–276). Jossey-Bass/Wiley.

Calancie, L., Frerichs, L., Davis, M. M., Sullivan, E., White, A. M., et al. (2021). Consolidated framework for collaboration research derived from a systematic review of theories, models, frameworks and principles for cross-sector collaboration. *PLoS One, 16*(1), e0244501. https://doi.org/10.1371/journal.pone.0244501

Coalition for Community Schools at the Institute for Educational Leadership. (2020). https://www.communityschools.org/. Retrieved 2 April, 2024.

Collaborative for Academic, Social and Emotional Learning. (2021, June). *The CASEL guide to schoolwide SEL essentials: A printable compilation of key activities and tools for school team*. CASEL – Guide to Schoolwide SEL. https://schoolguide.casel.org/uploads/sites/2/2019/09/2021.6.15_School-Guide-Essentials.pdf

Collins, E., Clark, M. A., & Taplan, D. H. (2016). *A pathway to well-being for children and families: Progress, plans and potential building bright futures*. ActKnowledge. January 2016. https://actknowledge.org/PDFs/BBFFinal1-20-16-2.pdf

Commonwealth Fund. (2023, January 31). U.S. health care from a global perspective, 2022: Accelerating spending, worsening outcomes. *Improving health care quality issue briefs*. Retrieved May 3, 2024, from https://www.commonwealthfund.org/publications/issue-briefs/2023/jan/us-health-care-global-perspective-2022

Covelli, L., Engberg, J., & Opper, I. M. (2022). *Leading indicators of long-term success in community schools: Evidence from New York City*. (EdWorkingPaper: 22-669). Retrieved from Annenberg Institute at Brown University 4 April 2024. https://doi.org/10.26300/59q2-ek65

Duncan, G. J., & Murnane, R. J. (2014, January). *Restoring opportunity: The crisis of inequality and the challenge for American education*. Harvard Education Press.

Durlak, J. A., Domitrovich, C. E., Weissberg, R. P., & Gullotta, T. P. (2015). *Handbook of social and emotional learning : Research and practice*. https://ci.nii.ac.jp/ncid/BB19322885

Ennis, G., & Tofa, M. (2019). Collective impact: A review of the peer-reviewed research. *Australian Social Work, 73*, 1–16. https://doi.org/10.1080/0312407X.2019.1602662

Forman, S. G., Olin, S. S., Hoagwood, K. E., Crowe, M., & Saka, N. (2009). Evidence-based interventions in schools: Developers' views of implementation barriers and facilitators. *School Mental Health, 1*(1), 26–36.

Galderisi, S., Heinz, A., Kastrup, M., Beezhold, J., & Sartorius, N. (2015). Toward a new definition of mental health. *World Psychiatry, 14*(2), 231–233. https://doi.org/10.1002/wps.20231PMID:26043341

Global Mind Project (2024, March 4). The Mental State of the World in 2023: A Perspective on Internet-Enabled Populations. Sapienlabs.org. Retrieved June 8, 2024, from The Mental State of the World in 2023 A Perspective on Internet-Enabled Populations

Hattie, J. (2008). *Visible learning: A synthesis of over 800 meta-analyses relating to achievement*. Routledge.

Kania, J., & Kramer, M. (2011). Collective impact. *Stanford Social Innovation Review (9), 1*(winter), 36–41.

Kania, J., Williams, J., Schmitz, P., Brady, S., Kramer, M., & Juster, J. S. (2022). Centering equity in collective impact. *Stanford Social Innovation Review (Winter)*, 38–45. https://ssir.org/articles/entry/centering_equity_in_collective_impact

Langley, A. K., Nadeem, E., Kataoka, S. H., Stein, B. D., & Jaycox, L. H. (2010). Evidence-based mental health programs in schools: Barriers and facilitators of successful implementation. *School Mental Health, 2*(3), 105–113. https://doi.org/10.1007/s12310-0109038-1

Le, L. K. D., Esturas, A. C., Mihalopoulos, C., Chiotelis, O., Bucholc, J., Chatterton, M. L., & Engel, L. (2021). Cost-effectiveness evidence of mental health prevention and promotion interventions: A systematic review of economic evaluations. *PLoS Medicine, 18*(5), e1003606. https://doi.org/10.1371/journal.pmed.1003606

Maier, A., Daniel, J., & Oakes, J. (2017). *Community schools as an effective school improvement strategy: A review of the evidence* (Research brief). Learning Policy Institute. Retrieved from https://learningpolicyinstitute.org/product/community-schools-effective-school-improvement-brief 10 May 2024

Marmot, M., Allen, J., Bell, R., Bloomer, E., Goldblatt, P., & Consortium for the European Review of Social Determinants of Health and the Health Divide. (2012). WHO European review of social determinants of health and the health divide. *Lancet (London, England), 380*(9846), 1011–1029. https://doi.org/10.1016/S0140-6736(12)61228-8

McGorry, P. D., Mei, C., Chanen, A., Hodges, C., Alvarez-Jimenez, M., & Killackey, E. (2022). Designing and scaling up integrated youth mental health care. *World psychiatry: Official journal of the World Psychiatric Association (WPA), 21*(1), 61–76. https://doi.org/10.1002/wps.20938

National Center for Safe, Supportive Learning Environments (NCSSF). (n.d.). *Implementing school mental health supports: Best practices in action*. Retrieved 30 Mar 2024, from https://safesupportivelearning.ed.gov/sites/default/files/13-ImpSchMnHlthSprtBtPrt-508_0.pdf

Panjwani, S., Graves-Boswell, T., & Flores, S. (2023). Evaluating collective impact initiatives: A systematic scoping review. *American Journal of Evaluation, 44*(3), 406–423. https://doi.org/10.1177/10982140221130266

Purkey, S. C., & Smith, M. S. (1983, March). Effective schools: A review. *The Elementary School Journal, 83*(4), 427–452.

Purpose Built Communities. (2024). Retrieved March 30, 2024, from https://purposebuiltcommunities.org

Rittel, H. W. J., & Webber, M. M. (1973). Dilemmas in a general theory of planning. *Policy Sciences, 4*, 155–169. https://doi.org/10.1007/BF01405730

Roussos, S. T., & Fawcett, S. B. (2000). A review of collaborative partnerships as a strategy for improving community health. *Annual Review of Public Health, 21*, 369–402. https://doi.org/10.1146/annurev.publhealth.21.1.369

U.S. Department of Education's Office of Elementary & Secondary Education. (2020). *Leveraging evidence-based practices for local school improvement*. Retrieved June 11, 2024, from https://oese.ed.gov/resources/oese-technical-assistance-centers/state-support-network/resources/leveraging-evidence-based-practices-local-school-improvement/

Wolff, T. (2016). Ten places where collective impact gets it wrong. *Global Journal of Community Psychology Practice, 7*(1), 1–11. Retrieved June 11, 2024, from https://www.gjcpp.org/pdfs/Tom%20Wolff%20Collective%20Impact%20critique-CopyeditFINAL.pdf

World Health Organization. (2004). *Promoting mental health: Concepts, emerging evidence, practice* (Summary report). World Health Organization.

World Health Organization. (2014). *Social determinants of health*. WHO.

Index

P. G. Bray, A. Maerlender (eds.), *Adolescent Public Mental Health*,
https://doi.org/10.1007/978-3-031-68294-0

GPSR Compliance

The European Union's (EU) General Product Safety Regulation (GPSR) is a set of rules that requires consumer products to be safe and our obligations to ensure this.

If you have any concerns about our products, you can contact us on ProductSafety@springernature.com

In case Publisher is established outside the EU, the EU authorized representative is:

Springer Nature Customer Service Center GmbH
Europaplatz 3
69115 Heidelberg, Germany

The manufacturer's authorised representative in the EU is Springer Nature Customer Service Centre GmbH, Europaplatz 3, 69115 Heidelberg, Germany. If you have any concerns regarding our products, please contact ProductSafety@springernature.com

Printed and bound by CPI Group (UK) Ltd, Croydon, CR0 4YY
01/10/2026
02225857-0003